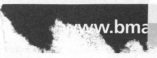
the**facts**

Huntington's
disease

the**facts**

Huntington's disease

SECOND EDITION

OLIVER QUARRELL
Consultant in Clinical Genetics
Sheffield Children's Hospital
Sheffield, UK

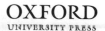

OXFORD
UNIVERSITY PRESS

OXFORD

UNIVERSITY PRESS

Great Clarendon Street, Oxford OX2 6DP

Oxford University Press is a department of the University of Oxford.
It furthers the University's objective of excellence in research, scholarship,
and education by publishing worldwide in

Oxford New York

Auckland Cape Town Dar es Salaam Hong Kong Karachi
Kuala Lumpur Madrid Melbourne Mexico City Nairobi
New Delhi Shanghai Taipei Toronto

With offices in

Argentina Austria Brazil Chile Czech Republic France Greece
Guatemala Hungary Italy Japan Poland Portugal Singapore
South Korea Switzerland Thailand Turkey Ukraine Vietnam

Oxford is a registered trade mark of Oxford University Press
in the UK and in certain other countries

Published in the United States
by Oxford University Press Inc., New York

© Oxford University Press, 2008

The moral rights of the author have been asserted
Database right Oxford University Press (maker)

First edition published 1999

British Library Cataloguing in Publication Data

Data available

Library of Congress Cataloguing in Publication Data

Data available

ISBN 978-0-19-921201-9 (Pbk.)

10 9 8 7 6 5 4 3 2 1

Typeset in Plantin
by Cepha Imaging Pvt. Ltd., Bangalore, India
Printed in Great Britain
on acid-free paper by
Ashford Colour Press, Gosport, Hampshire

Contents

Preface to the second edition

When I first wrote this book, my primary aim was to help you, the families, understand more about Huntington's disease. Of course, a secondary benefit was to help professionals with whom you come into contact at different stages of the illness. This remains the aim of the second edition. Publishing a second edition has given me the opportunity to update the clinical chapters and include quotes from others, which I hope makes the content more real for the intended audience. Some of the quotes are positive and uplifting, whereas others emphasize some of the difficulties that can be encountered.

It is nearly nine years since I wrote the first edition and nearly fifteen years since the gene for Huntington's disease and the protein, huntingtin, for which it is the code, were identified. There has been considerable research activity in that period involving laboratory scientists, clinicians, and families. Results from this research necessitate updating some of the basic scientific information. Both normal and abnormal huntingtin are involved in many processes within the cell. At present, we do not understand the early steps in the process by which some, but not all, cells are damaged by the abnormal huntingtin. I have tried to explain both the progress that has been made and some of the difficulties that have been encountered. Although there is frustration for families, scientists, and doctors that we do not have a treatment that delays the onset or slows nerve cell damage, research activity continues as a large multinational collaborative effort.

In preparing the second edition I have been helped by Helen Brewer from the Huntington's Disease Association, who read and commented on the chapters as they were revised. My colleague, Gerrit Dommeralt, from the

International Huntington Association, kindly provided the contact details of Huntington's disease organizations. I am grateful to Emma Marchant and Pete Stevenson at Oxford University Press for their help in modernizing and updating this little book. The patient quotes in Chapter 4 have been published in article Smith JA, Brewer HM, Etough V, Stanley CA, Glendinning NW, and Quarrell OW 2006. The personal experience of juvenile Huntington's disease: an interpretative phenomenological analysis of parents' accounts of the primary features of a rare genetic condition, *Clinical Genetics*, 69(6) 486-96. I am grateful to Dr. Elisabeth Rosser for information about the problems of testing young people for juvenile Huntington's disease. Two other contributions were by Brendan Stubbs, Physiotherapy Department, St Andrew's Health Care, Northants, and Andy Mantell, Social Studies Department, University of Chichester. Finally, updating this book required the direct encouragement and support of my wife, Gillian, and my sons, as well as tolerance for the time I spent away from the family.

Preface to the first edition

Huntington's disease poses lots of problems. Whether you have Huntington's disease, are caring for someone with Huntington's disease, or are at risk of developing the condition in the future, you are likely to have lots of questions. You may see a number of different professionals from time to time. Some of the more obvious professionals involved include: your local family doctor, a neurologist, a clinical geneticist, and possibly a psychiatrist. In addition, other professionals such as social workers, speech therapists, physiotherapists, nurses, and home helps are likely to be involved with your family. You may also come into contact with a patients' organization, either to obtain information, or to donate money or to attend meetings of local groups. You and your family may obtain help, support, and information from any or all of these sources at different times. One aim of this book is to supplement these various sources of information.

A second aim of this book is to give the reader a greater understanding of the problems involved in caring for relatives with Huntington's disease even though the solutions to these problems may be difficult to find. The first section of the book, Chapters 1–3, discusses some of the main medical facts. It is important to emphasize that, although patients with Huntington's disease have features in common, not everyone shows every aspect of the condition. Some carers have more problems with the physical aspect of the disease, whilst other families have more difficulty with the mental and personality changes that can occur. While there is no treatment to stop nerve cells in the brain dying early, there are ways to help families cope with some of the problems that occur. It is frustrating for families to realize that there is no magic cure for Huntington's disease; but doctors too are frustrated by not having the answers to all the problems.

Huntington's disease is a genetic condition. A third aim of this book is to explain how the identification of the gene has improved our knowledge and made available more options if you are at risk of developing Huntington's disease. Television programmes and newspapers frequently discuss the impact of genetic testing. Indeed, Huntington's disease is becoming more familiar to the general public, in part because of media stories, both factual and fictional. Chapter 4 concentrates on an explanation of the genetic aspects of the disorder and describes the story of cloning the gene. Nowadays, doctors offer genetic counselling to most families. Alternatively, families may take the initiative and ask for genetic counselling. Chapter 5 describes various aspects of genetic counselling. It is important to remember that although you will not always be offered genetic counselling, you do not have to attend straight away. It is perfectly acceptable to delay attending the genetic clinic until you are ready. Although you may discuss genetic tests with a counsellor, it is for you to decide if they are in your best interests.

A fourth aim of this little book is to consider prospects for the future. Chapter 7 describes the changes which occur in the brain; that leads on to a discussion of the latest research activity and ideas for future research.

Finally, patients' organizations play a prominent role in partnership with professionals, so Chapter 9 explains how these groups have developed in different countries.

Huntington's disease is a rare disorder and it is easy to think you are alone. In a town with a population of a quarter of a million, there will be approximately 18–25 patients diagnosed with Huntington's disease, but there will be many more people at risk of developing the condition, so it is a significant issue for a lot of people. The overall aim of this book is to give you more knowledge and understanding of Huntington's disease.

1

Facts and figures about Huntington's disease

Key points

♦ The first succinct description of the condition was given in 1872 by George Huntington.

♦ Approximately 1 person in 10,000 has Huntington's disease.

♦ Although Huntington's disease is rare, its genetic nature means it affects a large number of family members.

♦ It is difficult to date the onset of problems precisely, but in general the condition lasts for about 20 years.

Huntington's disease is a condition that affects the brain. Our brains contain millions of nerve cells, each one of which makes connections with many other nerve cells. We use our brains for thinking, planning, and remembering events, but the brain also controls a lot of processes automatically. The brain controls the movements of the body so that they are smooth and automatic. For example, when you wanted to pick up this book you were able to do so because your brain was able to co-ordinate a number of different functions without you giving each one conscious thought. We can consider some of the steps in this example: information from your eyes and where your hands were in relation to the book was co-ordinated; you could then smoothly move your arm so that your hand was close to the book; and you could use your fingers and thumb to pick up the book. All this movement was achieved without unbalancing the rest of your body.

The nerve cells in particular parts of the brain serve specific functions. In a person with Huntington's disease some nerve cells, in specific areas of the brain, die early. This produces a pattern of problems that allows doctors to make a diagnosis of Huntington's disease. We will consider this pattern of nerve cell loss in Chapter 9, but for the moment will continue with some of the more basic facts about Huntington's disease.

The history of Huntington's disease

Why is it called Huntington's disease?

Many medical conditions are named after a doctor who recognized and gave a clear description of the pattern of problems associated with that particular disorder. In our case Huntington's disease is named after an American doctor called George Huntington. Although George Huntington was not the first person to describe the condition, his was the first clear, succinct account. When other doctors then wanted to write about their patients they called the condition 'Huntington's chorea'. This now raises two questions.

What is 'chorea' and why has the name been changed to Huntington's disease?

A lot of medical terms are derived from either the Greek or Latin languages. The word 'chorea' comes from the Greek word for dance. Nowadays, it is a word used to describe unwanted involuntary movements. Some involuntary movements are useful, such as breathing or blinking, but a patient with Huntington's disease has movements of the face, body, and limbs that are random and purposeless. I will describe the various types of movement problems in more detail in the next chapter, but for now it is enough to say that chorea is the most frequent movement problem seen in Huntington's disease. Chorea is not the only movement disorder that can be recognized, and as the emotional and behavioural aspects can be more of a difficulty for the patient and the family, the term 'Huntington's disease' has become fashionable in recent times. As with any fashion it takes time for the change to be widely adopted, so it is possible that you will still hear the term 'Huntington's chorea'.

What was so remarkable about George Huntington's description?

George Huntington wrote a medical paper that was published in the Philadelphia-based *Medical and Surgical Reporter* in 1872. The title of the paper was 'On Chorea'. Huntington's disease is not the only cause of chorea, and at that time chorea was mostly commonly the result of a particular infection. Nowadays, we seldom see chorea due to infection, but that is another story. Most of George Huntington's paper was about the then most common cause of chorea. However, on the last page he described a hereditary form of chorea. His account of families with the hereditary form of chorea is very succinct and accurate, and it enabled other doctors to separate this cause of chorea from the others.

It may be interesting to take a slight diversion and comment on why George Huntington was in a position to know so much about Huntington's disease at such a young age. George's forebears had migrated from England to the east coast of America. His father and grandfather practised medicine in an area of Long Island, New York, and looked after families with this condition. George first met someone with the condition at the age of eight, when he travelled on medical rounds with his father. George qualified as a doctor and wrote his paper soon afterwards, while still only 21 years old. He was able to draw on his father's experiences of the condition and the original manuscript contains notes made by his father.

Other landmarks in the history of Huntington's disease

In the early part of the twentieth century there were relatively few publications on Huntington's disease, but the pattern of inheritance was confirmed. In addition, there were attempts to identify the number of patients in a given area, and some of the changes in the brain were documented. With time these studies became more sophisticated. The first book devoted to Huntington's disease was published by Michael Hayden in 1981. Although the book is based on his study of families with Huntington's disease in South Africa, it is clear that most of the natural history, basic genetics, and patterns of nerve cell damage in the brain have been well established.

Other notable landmarks include the foundation of the lay organization called the Committee to Combat Huntington's Disease, which was founded in the USA by Marjorie Guthrie in 1967. Her husband, the folk singer Woodie Guthrie, had died of the condition that year. The development of organizations for patients and families is described in more detail in Chapter 12.

The struggle to identify the problem with the gene that causes Huntington's disease covered the period from the 1980s to 1993 and will be described in Chapter 5. The identification of the genetic mistake has helped remove some uncertainties about the diagnosis and has allowed the development of reliable predictive tests, but was never an end in itself. The objective was, and remains, to understand Huntington's disease so that effective treatments may be developed to alter its natural history or delay its onset. Apart from humans, no other animal develops Huntington's disease. Once the gene that causes it was identified, an important landmark was its insertion into laboratory animals. There are a number of animal and cellular models of Huntington's disease. Our understanding of Huntington's disease is summarized in Figure 1.1.

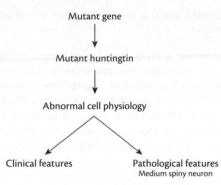

Mutant gene

↓

Mutant huntingtin

↓

Abnormal cell physiology

Clinical features   Pathological features
                           Medium spiny neuron

Figure 1.1 Summary of our understanding of Huntington's disease. It is possible to tell a coherent story about the mistake in the gene which produces an abnormal protein. How this damages particular cells in the brain is still unclear. It is also possible to describe the clinical features seen in Huntington's disease and the changes that take place in the brain.

Genes are the instructions to make proteins. Knowledge of the Huntington's disease gene allowed the identification of the protein for which it is the code. The protein was called huntingtin. Abnormal huntingtin results in abnormal cellular processes; in turn, this leads to the clinical features that families and doctors recognize. Our knowledge of how these abnormal cellular processes leads to Huntington's disease is incomplete. A lot of progress has been made, but so far a treatment to alter the natural history is unavailable. For now, I want to concentrate on the numbers of people affected and some aspects of the natural history of the disease.

How many people are affected?

In order to answer this question a doctor has to define a reasonable area, count the number of patients with Huntington's disease who were alive on a particular date, and compare that with the number of healthy people alive at the same time. This seems simple enough, but there are a number of problems with this type of study. Defining a reasonable area is important; if the area is too small then the result can be very misleading. If we take a row of houses that contain ten people and one person has Huntington's disease, then 1 person in 10 has Huntington's disease—but this answer is absurd. If the area is too large, then it may be difficult to identify all the patients with Huntington's disease. The early studies tended to underestimate the number of Huntington's disease patients. If we look at a number of studies of numbers of patients in the UK that have been done in the last thirty years or so, then it is clear that results ranged between 4 and 10 patients with Huntington's disease for every 100,000 of the population. Some studies are more sophisticated than others so a convenient estimate would be 7–10 patients per 100,000. This means that in the UK, which has a population of approximately 60 million, there are about 4,200–6000 patients with Huntington's disease at any one time. It is now easy to see that Huntington's disease is a rare disorder, but if we count the carers and close relatives of a patient then many more people are affected by it. In addition, a patient has Huntington's disease for a very long period of time, so the condition represents a significant problem.

Huntington's disease in various parts of the world

It is reasonable to ask if Huntington's disease occurs in all parts of the world and if different countries or continents have different numbers of Huntington's disease patients, and if so why? As we started with the UK it may be interesting to note that studies suggest very similar numbers of people are affected in European countries.

We can now go on to consider the English-speaking nations, since they were largely founded by migration from the UK and other parts of Europe. As might be expected, the number of people affected by Huntington's disease is again in the range of 4–10 per 100,000 in Canada, the USA, and Australia. It is also interesting to ask if Huntington's disease affects the native populations. This type of information is more difficult to gather. It may be that there are fewer cases among these peoples, but detailed studies have not been undertaken. Studies of numbers of patients with Huntington's disease have not been done in the Indian subcontinent; however, there has been a study of Huntington's disease among the immigrant population in the UK, which gave a result of 1.75 per 100,000. There are a number of reasons why this figure could be an underestimate, so it is reasonable to assume that Huntington's disease does occur in India and that if it were possible to do a systematic study, the numbers of people affected could be similar to that seen in Europe. Similarly, detailed studies have not been undertaken in other parts of Asia, but it has been well documented that there are fewer cases in Japan than in Europe.

Interesting things happen if relatively few people migrate to a sparsely populated part of the world. If one of the founders of that population has Huntington's disease and goes on to have a lot of descendants then the number of people affected with Huntington's disease can become unusually high. This has happened in Tasmania (Australia) and has also happened in an area of Venezuela.

One large family that lives around the shores of Lake Maracaibo in Venezuela has been particularly important in the search for the Huntington's disease gene. This story will be told in more detail in Chapter 5.

When does Huntington's disease start?

This question gives the impression that the age of onset of Huntington's disease can be documented accurately. This is not so. A person does not go to bed healthy and wake up the next day with Huntington's disease. Many people at risk for Huntington's disease have asked me to describe how Huntington's disease starts. On the face of it this is a reasonable question, but in fact it is difficult to give a clear answer. The problem is that some of the early features of Huntington's disease can occur in anyone. When doctors make a diagnosis of any condition they are effectively recognizing a pattern. The problem comes when a patient starts with mood changes or being less tidy than they once were. This can occur in anyone, and it is only possible to estimate that this was the start of Huntington's disease when more obvious signs, such as abnormal movements, occur later on.

Someone experienced in seeing patients with Huntington's disease may recognize small abnormal movements as chorea, especially if there is a family history. However, many patients will not see an experienced doctor at this time, and it may be some years before the patient and members of the family recognize that there is a problem and seek medical help. If the doctor then asks how long they have had a problem, the family have some difficulty in remembering the start because the condition comes on slowly. They may be able to give an estimate of the start, but it will not be accurate. For this reason, the onset of Huntington's disease is best described as insidious. As some of the very early changes can be non-specific, an experienced doctor who happens to see someone around this time may have some suspicions, but will want to examine the patient again to see if the signs persist and gradually worsen over time.

As we will see in Chapter 5, the identification of the gene has resulted in people at risk of developing Huntington's disease coming for predictive tests. As someone who offers predictive testing, I sometimes see people who have very minimal chorea and I am able to make a diagnosis much earlier than would have happened before these tests were available. In the past, the patient and family would have waited longer before seeing a doctor.

Despite these limitations, it has been possible to summarize the age of onset of patients in the form of a graph (Fig. 1.2). Over the years there have been a number of studies estimating the age of onset of Huntington's disease, but they all result in an S-shaped graph like this one. Given the shape of this graph,

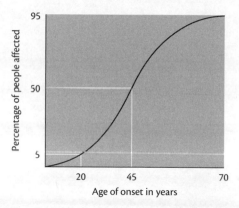

Figure 1.2 Age of onset curve for Huntington's disease. Huntington's disease can develop at almost any age but most people develop the condition between the ages of 35 and 55 years.

it is easy to work out that Huntington's disease can start at almost any age, but most people develop the condition between the ages of 35 and 55 years.

How long does Huntington's disease last?

Again, this is a very simple question but one that is difficult to answer accurately. In a study of patients with Huntington's disease in a particular area it is possible to know precisely when an affected person died. The problem comes in trying to estimate when that person started to have Huntington's disease. As we saw in the last section, it is possible to ask the family to give an estimate but it will not be absolutely precise. A number of studies have accepted this limitation and estimated the duration of the disease. The results have varied but an average of 15–16 years is a reasonable estimate. Of course you have to remember that this is only an average, so some patients will have had the condition for a longer and some for a shorter time. Given the difficulties of families accurately dating the onset of the condition, I prefer to think of Huntington's disease as a condition which lasts around twenty years.

Figure 4.2 ...

How long does Huntington's disease last?

2

The physical features of Huntington's disease

> ## ➲ Key points
>
> ◆ The physical features change over time.
>
> ◆ Chorea usually starts early but slowing of movements occurs and may become more obvious as the condition progresses.
>
> ◆ Problems with balance are difficult to solve.
>
> ◆ Difficulties occur with speech and swallowing.
>
> ◆ The type of professional help required changes as someone goes through the different stages of the illness.
>
> ◆ As time goes by, it is important that the family carer can also care for themselves.

As we saw in the last chapter, Huntington's disease (HD) lasts for a long time so it may be that you or your family can relate to only part of what is written here. In order to break up the story I have arbitrarily divided the description of a typical person into early, middle, and late stages. Let us first consider the problems of someone starting with Huntington's disease in middle age; we can then consider some of the features seen in people with particularly early onset or particularly late onset. Huntington's disease can start with either physical problems, changes in personality or both. In some people the personality changes can occur well before neurological signs are obvious. However, in this chapter I want to concentrate on the physical aspects of the condition.

What are the physical signs in the early stages of Huntington's disease?

Some people are aware of Huntington's disease in the family and suspect problems early. On the other hand, as Huntington's disease develops slowly, some people may not notice problems or ignore them for a very long time. One of the earliest physical signs of the disease is **chorea**, or involuntary movements. It is very hard to explain the difference between chorea and simple fidgeting. When families ask me to point out what I see as chorea I sometimes ask them to describe a particular colour, such as green. As you might expect I often get the answer that grass is green. This allows me to go on and explain that most people cannot easily define 'green', but they have no difficulty in pointing out objects which are green. The same applies to the recognition of chorea by professionals and family members who have seen it regularly. In the early stages of the disease these extra movements occur infrequently and are not especially large. They are different from a fidgety movement, but I find it difficult to describe this in words. Chorea is usually considered as an involuntary movement, but patients with Huntington's disease also have problems with voluntary movement. At this stage of the illness, the movements may not trouble the patient and sometimes they are not really noticed by the family.

The problems with voluntary movement are often very subtle in the early stages of the disorder and are best described as a slowing of movements. The technical term for this is **bradykinesia**. A doctor may specifically look for signs of slowing of movements by asking you to flick your eyes from one side to the other very rapidly. These eye movements are normally very rapid, but in someone with Huntington's disease it is possible to detect changes in the way they are performed. Other similar tests involve asking you to perform rapid alternating movements such as flicking the tongue from side to side or tapping your index finger and thumb together very rapidly.

Balance is a difficult problem in Huntington's disease, so a doctor may also check the way you walk and may even ask you to take a number of steps putting the heel of one foot against the toe of the other (heel to toe walking).

The speech of someone with Huntington's disease can become slurred and for this reason a person may be asked to repeat certain syllables, which can detect subtle changes. It is important to realize that subtle changes in each of these tests can occur in a large number of conditions other than Huntington's disease but that it is the *pattern* of abnormalities that allows a diagnosis to be made. In the early stages, not many physical signs may be present. They may be confined to chorea, which is more obvious when you are stressed, some slowing of eye movements, and minor problems in other areas of the clinical examination.

Surprisingly, these are not often major problems for the person affected, although they clearly indicate that the disease has started. Many people are able to continue with their job for some time. It would be extremely unlikely that any drugs would be considered for the movement disorder at this stage. In fact, physical problems may be less important than difficulties with memory, emotion or behaviour; these will be discussed in the next chapter. I have already made the point that the onset of Huntington's disease is insidious. Figure 2.1 shows the time course of the disease and the time when you might seek medical help. Exactly what is said to a particular person (or couple) will depend on when, during the course of the disease, you see a specialist and on what type of question you are asking. If you come and say that you think Huntington's disease has started then it is relatively easy to answer you sympathetically but directly. On the other hand, I frequently see people in the clinic in whom signs of Huntington's disease are present but who are completely unaware of them. If this is the case, it may be more appropriate for a doctor to get to know these patients over a few appointments before voicing suspicions that the disease has actually started.

Some families have complained to me that once a diagnosis of Huntington's disease is made they feel abandoned afterwards by the medical profession. I can understand how these feelings arise, since it may be that nothing specific is required for a number of years. My own practice is to leave it up to the person or family concerned whether they want to come to the clinic once a year or wait until they feel it is necessary. An alternative to being seen in the clinic is to contact your own local doctor. In some countries, patients' organizations

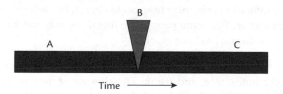

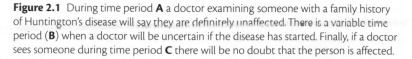

Figure 2.1 During time period **A** a doctor examining someone with a family history of Huntington's disease will say they are definitely unaffected. There is a variable time period (**B**) when a doctor will be uncertain if the disease has started. Finally, if a doctor sees someone during time period **C** there will be no doubt that the person is affected.

(which are discussed in more detail in Chapter 12) have a network of available contacts.

Another important point to come from this description is that if none of these signs are seen in people at risk of Huntington's disease, they can be reassured that the disease has not yet started. Some people at risk are able to put the issue to the back of their minds, whereas others look for signs of the disorder. It is important to realize that a doctor does not rely on recognizing one particular sign to make the diagnosis, but on a pattern.

What about driving?

This can be a very sensitive issue for some people. In the UK the rule is clear: you have to inform the Driver and Vehicle Licensing Agency (DVLA) if you have a medical condition that affects your fitness as a driver. There are several reasons why you may find this difficult: first, you have to have accepted the diagnosis in your own mind, and secondly, it is difficult to contemplate the possible loss of easy mobility. Given that the features of Huntington's disease slowly worsen, it is almost inevitable that you will have to rely on someone else to drive you at some stage. The real difficulty is deciding when this stage has been reached. It is often better if you inform the licensing authority yourself rather than get into a position where this decision is forced on you. People who are in the early stages of the disease are sometimes given licences that can be reviewed on a regular basis.

What are the physical problems in the middle stages of the disease?

The term 'middle stages of the disease' is very imprecise, but it covers a long period of time when the condition has worsened so that the movements are obvious. If you are at this stage then you will probably no longer be working and will have difficulty performing household chores, but will still have quite a lot of independence. For some people the diagnosis may not be made until this stage of the disease has been reached.

The chorea may be very obvious, with relatively large movements of the muscles of the limbs, face, and trunk. The slowing of movements will have worsened, but perhaps will still be masked by the chorea. For some people the movements are a problem, but frequently the social, emotional, and behavioural problems are more of a concern to the family. At this stage people may complain of problems with balance. Patients with Huntington's disease do fall, but I have always been struck by the fact that the falls are relatively infrequent, given that the choreic movements are obvious.

It is possible to give drugs to slow down the movements, but this requires some thought. If drugs are given that reduce the chorea then it is likely that they will make the other movement disorders of bradykinesia and dystonia (see below) worse. Drugs may need to be given to help with the emotional and behavioural problems, but these drugs also have an effect on the movement. A reasonable approach is to say that there is no medicine that will stop the nerve cells dying, but treatment is available to help with some of the problems this causes. A doctor, in discussion with the person and his or her relatives, has to decide the main issue for everyone concerned and not treat the movements in isolation.

During this stage of the disease your speech is likely to become more obviously slurred. In addition, difficulties with swallowing may also become apparent. These difficulties affect all aspects of the swallowing process, including taking an appropriate portion of food and chewing it fully. A referral to a speech therapist and a dietician can be useful to give advice to the carer about some practical issues, including how to deal with choking episodes.

It is during the middle stage that you and your family may want to discuss how you would like the later stages of the disease to be managed. This is a difficult and sensitive issue, but once you have done this with your family you can discuss options with your doctor. A lot of patients develop pneumonia as the very last stage of the condition. If you have strong views that you do not want a lot of treatment with antibiotics at that time then you can discuss the option of leaving an advance directive. Some people are treated with a feeding tube, which is placed through the tummy directly into the stomach. This is not always necessary, but again it may be helpful to discuss the option well in advance so that you have an opportunity to express your views on this and if necessary record them.

What physical problems occur in the later stages of the disease?

As the disease progresses, **dystonia** may become apparent. This term is used to describe the fact that the limbs can be held in unusual positions. At this time there is a mixture of movement problems, consisting of chorea, bradykinesia, and dystonia. Exactly what is seen in any one person depends on the exact mixture of these problems. Generally speaking, the chorea tends to level off but the bradykinesia and dystonia worsen. In some cases, as the disease progresses, the person appears stiff and **rigid**.

Being a carer

There are issues about caring for someone with Huntington's disease in the early and middle stages. Although there are physical problems at these stages, I think more of the care is around managing the emotional and behavioural problems, which are discussed in the next chapter. This section concentrates on some of the problems that may be encountered in the later stages. Some readers may not be ready to think about the later stages; if so, you can skip over this section.

Although the term 'later stages' is arbitrary, I am assuming that the person with Huntington's disease has reached the stage of needing a lot of physical care, such as help with dressing, feeding, and going to the toilet. This care may be provided in an institution, such as a nursing home, or at home. There is a problem with having a section on being a carer in a description of the later stages: care is required at all stages, although the type of care varies. In the next chapter, I will deal with some of the behavioural aspects, which may be more important than the physical problems at earlier stages of the illness.

If you are caring for someone at home then it is important to ensure that arrangements are made for you to care for yourself. You should not feel guilty for needing some time of your own. It may be that help from other family members is available. Unfortunately, the amount of professional help provided varies from place to place, but regular respite care may be a way forward. Behavioural difficulties often occur alongside physical problems, so getting the affected person to accept the need for respite care can be a real problem. In addition, respite care can be provided at home. Continuity of arrangements is important. My own practice is to encourage the involvement of social services early on so that support mechanisms are in place before a crisis develops. Whatever solution you reach, remember that as a carer you also need care and support. It may be at this time that you want to talk to other people in a similar situation, in which case you can attend meetings of the Huntington's Disease Association or other local support groups.

I have the opportunity to quote some information given to me by family members and other professionals. I have included some of these conversations below with minimal alterations. Although there is a pattern to Huntington's disease, each person is different. I have decided to keep both positive and negative comments. I hope that you and your family may be able to relate to some if not all of these comments.

ℹ Patient's perspective

I am indebted to one particular couple for commenting on their different perspectives of the diagnosis of Huntington's disease and its implications for them over the years. Attending the pre-diagnosis counselling together over a period of approximately six months led to two very different responses. The husband was the patient. When the diagnosis was confirmed his reaction was relief, with the comment, "I'm not going mad then".

"My husband's strong personality and his need to know and understand problems and solve them (as best we humans can) based on factual information enabled him to view this diagnosis in a positive light. He could now get to grips with how he would deal with the future. He felt positive and in control of the situation."

His wife and carer's response to the diagnosis confirmation was bewilderment, resulting in denial:

"Bombarded with information, some relevant to that time, much with a view to the long term. Information which made me feel negative (depressed) and I found it impossible to associate the discussions with medical professionals regarding all aspects of HD with my wonderful husband."

Denial

"Irrationally over a long period of time I felt everything would be OK if I tried/worked harder to keep life together 'as normal' whatever that is! Feeling guilty for not being able to control the illness. Working harder and harder, exhausted most of the time, denial comes with a cost."

Letting go of denial

"Gradually becoming more assertive and much stronger enabled me to organize and obtain the correct care for my husband. Liaison with all levels of medical professionals as many aspects of medical assistance have been required during our HD journey. Genetics and neurology consultations, HD outreach nurse, speech therapist, dietician, occupational therapist, physiotherapist, to name but a few. There were routine hospital appointments plus many professionals visiting our home on a regular basis.

The greatest gift any carer can make is to be able to give practical support, liaising with all professionals to enable the best possible care for your loved one. I have been the link between my husband and the service providers. Being in control of the situation takes away the negative feelings and gives more positives. *Situations along the way are stressful—ask for help and, importantly, accept help.*

I am the only person who can give the emotional support to my husband and enjoy together all that's made us a couple over a very long time and continue to celebrate our relationship."

ⓘ Patient's perspective

I am indebted to a family member of an HD patient who sent me these notes about being a carer and agreed to have them published anonymously. Your experiences may be different but I hope you can relate to some of the points being made.

"**Aim**: To ensure my wife has the best possible time for the remainder of her life.

Objective: At the end of each day I will be able to say at least one thing that we have enjoyed doing."

Balancing HD and life

"Keeping HD in perspective is a challenge. HD dominates my life to the point where I need to remind myself to carry on living. All the professionals I meet focus on their area of expertise and most on problems in this area. So any contact with them tends to leave me feeling negative; what I need to do is to balance this against how my wife is doing overall.

So, yes, HD is a part of our lives and needs to be balanced against what I am doing to achieve my objective."

My role

"I am the expert on my wife and the person who in all senses of the word cares for her. Everyone else is a bit player who may be able to help me achieve my objective. I need to orchestrate them to ensure her needs are met."

Looking for the options

"Stress for me is feeling that I have no control over my life and that of my wife. So actively searching for the choices I have at each turn is constructive. Even with HD symptoms there are choices, medication, counselling care aids, professional advice, etc."

HD: problem/opportunity

"Yes, HD is a big problem but amazingly even this can be used to advantage. I took a redundancy deal from work. I used HD as an excuse; the fact was I was ready to leave and HD gave me the excuse.

My wife always wanted to travel so while she was well enough we travelled. We made a list of all the places she wanted to go to then slowly ticked them off; it felt great. So we used HD as the excuse to do or buy all the stuff we wanted to."

Routines

"Getting into a routine has proved a great way for me to help my wife. For example, every morning we go out somewhere: garden centres, shops, anywhere. The choice of where we go is my wife's—great! I don't have to think about that and my wife goes where she wants to. The important thing is it helps achieve my objective and my wife needs to think about it.

On a similar basis, she has a bath every night: the routine here helps with the personal hygiene issues."

Memories

"When my wife or I get really fed up I get the holiday photos out. I have them on disc now so she can view them on the television. We always feel a little better reminding ourselves that we have been to such interesting places. I guess all holiday pictures are great as they recall good times.

I also show the video of our son's graduation where we were so proud of him."

Positive feedback

"Acknowledging my wife's achievements is essential for me to achieve the objective. I am proud of how well she is dealing with HD and I tell her. To me it is part of a positive cycle.

I am happy talking to happy people but keep my wife away from negative people. I believe like attracts like."

Dealing with professional help

"I remind myself they are all bit players, and that she is a woman who happens to have HD.

Most professionals will give us ten minutes of their time; what I do to ensure this is used most effectively is give them a few pages of notes I have produced on the word processor. This is good for me as it means I don't have to struggle to remember things—good for them as they have a record and can focus. This gives more time on my wife.

To be honest it also makes me feel I am doing a more professional job as a carer and project this image to people I need to help me."

Information

"I find there is a mass of information available to help. The challenge is finding it and organizing it. On the computer I have the Google news alerts for HD, which produces at least five emails a day. It's interesting to see how drug companies view the opportunity to make money and the medical world's fascination with HD. The Huntington's Disease Association has a site; there are also chat rooms that I have found helpful. My problem is that I find it depressing to read details of the condition, so I don't do it. I only read what I believe will help.

I have an A4 folder with sections to help me access information; these include the district nurse, wheelchair service, social services, neurologist, Disability Living Allowance (DLA) etc."

Support available

"I work on the basis that anyone who helps me achieve my objective is my friend. These have included the GP, district nurse, rehabilitation team, consultants, and social services."

Time out

"My wife sleeps more and more; this is a change that is giving me time out to do things I enjoy, e.g. reading, gardening, DIY, etc. This enables me to function better and achieve the objective."

I'm OK

"For me HD is like a bereavement and requires a massive mental effort to deal with. Dealing with bereavement as with any change can be considered as a process with four stages: denial, acceptance, planning, then action.

Denial is pretending it will not happen, or some major breakthrough will occur with medical research. I have found that if I put too much effort into reading the research and news about HD I can raise my hopes and forget to focus on my objective. I still harbour the hope that a better treatment will be available, or better still a cure. But realistically, this will happen too late for my wife. This is me overcoming my denial.

Acceptance has been the most difficult for me and I am working at it all the time. My wife seems to be in front of me all the time, I guess because she lives each change whereas I just observe it. So the expression I use now is 'I am OK with my new role', even though it's not all right.

Planning is clearly writing the objective.

Action is working to achieve my objective."

Confirmation of objective achieved

"At the end of day when I tuck my wife in bed I recall all the things we have enjoyed doing. She normally repeats them back to me.

So this is confirmation of a good day and objective achieved.

On such nights I sleep well."

If the person with Huntington's disease is not very mobile, specially adapted chairs are available that help to prevent accidents due to the involuntary movements. One such chair, the Kirton™ chair, is shown in Figure 2.2. A physiotherapist may be involved at this stage to give advice about trying to maintain the best posture so as to avoid problems in the future. Other adaptations to the home have to be considered. It is not easy to be specific because individual needs and circumstances vary, but practical solutions should be sought. This is when the advice of an occupational therapist can be particularly important.

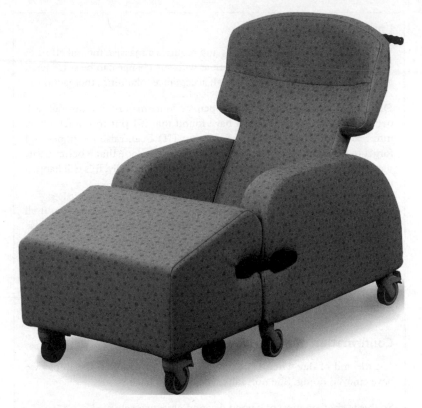

Figure 2.2 A number of chairs are available for someone in the later stages of Huntington's disease. They are padded to protect the person and are easy to keep clean. The leg rest can be removed to help with mobility and care. In addition a sheepskin cover can be used to help pressure areas. This photograph was kindly supplied by Kirton Healthcare™.

There may be problems with incontinence. It should not be assumed that the incontinence is always due to Huntington's disease, so it is useful to check first that an infection is not present. However, in the majority of cases, practical solutions such as pads, closeness to the toilet, and regular toileting have to be considered as well as the use of easily removed clothes. Help and advice may be obtained from district nursing services.

📄 Case study

(I am grateful to a physiotherapist colleague, Brendon Stubbs, for this vignette. It shows that even in the later stages of the condition it is still possible to help improve the comfort and quality of life of someone with a lot of physical problems.)

David had not had any physiotherapy input. He was unable to walk and was seated in a tilt-in-space chair that was in the reclined position. He also had soft-tissue shortening of muscles in his legs. David's neck was side-flexed to the right and this was uncomfortable for him. Nursing staff had been particularly concerned about his rigidity and explained they were having difficulty with moving him between the bed and the chair. Following the physiotherapy assessment, staff were advised not to recline David back in his chair as he had good unsupported sitting balance and so did not need this. This new position also had the added benefit that David could now see and interact with his environment. A neck support was provided to try to prevent further deterioration of posture. David received regular physiotherapy to mobilize the neck and help the muscles relax. A course of injections began to reduce the tension in the muscles. David's neck began to improve. He was now able to have it placed in midline; this helped to improve his trunk symmetry, and maintaining an upright posture became less effortful. Mealtimes became easier and less of a risk, as David had previously been choking regularly despite having food designed to help with this problem.

David had previously been given little opportunity to stand during the day; a schedule was co-ordinated with nursing staff to ensure David stood up at least every hour. Standing helps to maintain digestion and strong muscles and bones, and prevents soft-tissue shortening. Nursing staff were advised on how to facilitate David to stand. This regular exercise helped with transfers between bed and chair and these became easier. David's mood improved and standing regularly gave him the opportunity to feel more involved and active during the day.

David began to attend a weekly hydrotherapy session, which helped with relaxation, stretching of shortened muscles, and standing practice. David was also seen three times a week to do passive stretches to prevent contractures developing.

🄘 Patients' perspectives

The quotes below were given to me by Andy Mantell, who undertook a research project interviewing thirty-one family members who provided care. Where he has illustrated his points with quotes from patients, names have been changed to protect their identity.

The following strategies were identified by family members as ways they tried to cope with caring. Some were successful and some were not; in part this related to the type of person they were.

Live for today, plan for tomorrow

Some relatives gained control over difficult circumstances by planning for tomorrow. They tended to gain as much information as possible about HD in order to anticipate and ameliorate potential problems. This approach enabled them to direct rather than react to circumstances. In turn, this can reduce the number of crises that occur. It can enable the person with HD to have more of a say in their care and in what happens if they are no longer able to receive care at home.

However, reality often doesn't go to plan, as Tom observed:

"There were no strategies, no plan, you don't think 'Oh, how am I going to deal with it the next day.' You're so busy dodging bullets."

For others such as Tara it was too distressing to plan for the future because it meant facing losses to come:

"I don't like to think what the future may hold. I take one day at a time, I get up and just try and get through the day. If it's been a good day, good, and if it's been a bad day, then tomorrow might be better. And that's how really I've coped with it."

Relatives spoke of maintaining normality; this served to protect both them and the person with HD from facing the future. It also avoided unnecessary distress over possible symptoms to come; for example, not all people with HD develop aggressive behaviour.

Sustaining normality also served a therapeutic role for the person with HD. It ensured that their world remained familiar and predictable and served to try to preserve their role within that world as long as possible:

"We always said 'We've got a lot of living to do today and tomorrow.' You don't change today or tomorrow. You only change over a period of time if you don't keep doing things. So we have tried to maintain that we can do things." (Tracy)

Routine

Relatives found routine enabled both them and the person with HD to predict and manage their day and helped to sustain a sense of normality. This also worked well with involvement by care workers. However, some relatives missed being able to act spontaneously.

Keeping perspective

Relatives could find it difficult in their isolation to maintain a sense of perspective:

"Sometimes I think, am I imagining all this, blowing up all these problems out of proportion? And you just wonder, how much have I adjusted to the illness and the way she is behaving? That actually she's behaving quite abnormally but it seems normal to me, you know?" (Henry)

Maintaining a sense of perspective, for example through humour, prevented relatives from feeling overwhelmed. Having time to themselves, such as through respite, was seen as important to enable family members to take stock and re-evaluate their perspective:

"You step, you step back and first you do a damage assessment, on yourself, almost, you think 'Well, am I still intact, do things work?'" (Tom)

Attitude

Relatives spoke of the need to maintain a positive mental attitude in order to stay motivated:

"I think what I got my strength from is everything boils downs to Huntington's disease and I say: 'This thing isn't going to defeat me.' You cannot let it sweep over you. You must fight it; you've got to be strong in your mind." (Bob)

Most relatives talked about how they had changed the way they responded to the person with HD. This ranged from increased tolerance and patience to avoiding confrontations and secrecy. This was not necessarily due to fear of aggressive behaviour, as Henry explained:

"And I often think when the time is right at home to talk about it, when my wife is in a good mood, you don't actually want to spoil it by suddenly talking about Huntington's or some problem in the home."

In contrast, assertiveness was considered by relatives to be important to help keep the person with HD safe but also meet their own needs. Assertiveness was particularly employed where there was a conflict of interest and at times to try to gain control where the person with HD appeared to be out of control. It could, however, be very difficult to sustain in the face of aggression from the person with HD:

"So I tried to sort of tell him the truth, but then to be honest there's always a fear at the back of your mind that he's going to go into one. Might throw a wobbly." (Trudy)

Physical intervention

Some relatives found that they had to restrain the person with Huntington's disease, and some admitted that they had assaulted them:

"I might be either doing the, preparing the meal, or I might be washing up and he'd come and give you a punch in the back. And I'm sorry to say that I used to retaliate, because I used to turn round and I used to punch him." (Clare)

Others fled to protect themselves. In this group of relatives none withdrew completely but violence was one of the catalysts for the person with HD entering a care home.

Seeking help

Relatives were reluctant to seek help. When they did, it tended to be from friends and family before reluctantly turning to social services. Admission to care appeared to be influenced by emotional responses at times of crisis rather than proactive planning. All of the relatives had had contact from social services, but many recognized that they would have benefited from greater support sooner.

Weight loss

A characteristic feature of Huntington's disease is weight loss. A full explanation for this is not available, but it occurs in most patients. Part of the care may involve providing high-calorie food supplements. Occasionally feeding tubes are used in the later stage of the disease, but the decision to use a feeding tube has to take into account the overall condition of the person with Huntington's disease, together with any views that have previously been expressed and the wishes of the family.

Long-term care

So far I have assumed that the person with Huntington's disease is being looked after at home. Individual circumstances vary, so at some stage you may have to give some thought to a long-term stay in a nursing home or similar establishment. Whilst the need to do this may eventually become obvious, it is not something that is done easily or lightly. If you have been caring for a loved one then it may be natural to feel a little guilty if and when the time for long-term care arises. Finding a suitable nursing home may not be easy, but your local support group may be able to give advice and information based on experience.

It has not been possible to describe all the practical problems that can occur or comment on possible solutions. However, Table 2.1 summarizes the role of the various professional and lay groups that may be involved in care.

Table 2.1 Professionals and agencies involved in the care of someone with Huntington's disease

Professional or agency	Reason for involvement
Speech therapists and dieticians	Communication, swallowing problems, and nutrition
Occupational therapists and physiotherapists	Mobility, activities of daily living, and posture
District nurses	Incontinence and personal care
Social workers	Benefits and local care facilities, both respite and longer-term
Family doctor	Relevant medication, support, and referral to other professionals
Local support group	Support of the carer and information about local facilities
Specialist clinic	General support, relevant medication, and referral to other agencies

What are the features when Huntington's disease starts late in life?

In Chapter 4, I discuss features that are seen when the age of onset is very young (less than 20 years). At the other end of the spectrum from early onset is Huntington's disease starting late in life. As might be expected, the chorea tends to be more prominent and slowness and stiffness are less prominent. Superficially, the disease appears less disabling than when the onset is in mid-life or earlier. If Huntington's disease occurs late in life it is likely to be more difficult to establish a family history because the person's parents may have died many years previously, perhaps before they themselves showed signs of the condition. Chorea can be caused by conditions other than Huntington's disease, and a new genetic test has helped to resolve some difficult diagnoses. This is discussed again in Chapter 6. Not unreasonably, children of an elderly person with Huntington's disease may think that a late age of onset runs in the family. Whilst there is some statistical evidence for this, it is not reliable enough to give practical information to the children, as we shall see on page 62.

3

Behavioural and emotional aspects of Huntington's disease

> **➔ Key points**
>
> ◆ Changes in the brain result in problems with mood and thinking that cause behavioural problems.
>
> ◆ The behavioural problems may be more difficult to manage than the physical aspects.
>
> ◆ Depression is the most frequent mood change.
>
> ◆ Problems with thinking include difficulty switching between tasks and changing plans in the light of new information. This may result in outbursts of temper.
>
> ◆ The person with Huntington's disease cannot change easily so the carers and family have to make changes to avoid difficulties.

A doctor or scientist giving a brief description of Huntington's disease will say that it has three components: a **movement disorder**, impaired **cognition** (thinking), and a disturbance of **affect** (mood). The movement disorder was described in the last chapter; but now I want to concentrate on cognitive or thinking problems and difficulties with affect or mood.

We should not be surprised that behavioural and emotional problems, together with psychiatric illnesses, are associated with Huntington's disease. The brain has a limited number of ways of coping with a variety of stresses. Nowadays, there is much more openness about mental illness in newspapers and on television, so we know that many people become depressed, or mentally unwell, at some point in their lives. Someone with Huntington's disease has lost some nerve cells from the brain, so it is reasonable to suppose that an effect of this will be problems with behaviour and mental well-being.

I have indicated that many families find it more difficult to cope with the wide range of behavioural and emotional problems than the physical aspects of the condition. If you are caring for someone with Huntington's disease you can find these aspects are often very frustrating. As Huntington's disease lasts such a long time, and as each person is an individual, it is not possible to give a description that fits everybody. A further problem is that in some people it can be hard to disentangle problems related to a depressed mood from those due to impaired thinking and apathy.

Some of what follows may be familiar to you from your experiences of Huntington's disease, but I want to emphasize that not everyone gets everything. Another important point to highlight is that the problems in Huntington's disease are selective. This theme of selective problems is taken up again in later chapters when we consider which nerve cells are damaged by Huntington's disease, but it is helpful to know that not all aspects of thinking are damaged.

What are the main problems?

The majority of carers to whom I have spoken recognize descriptions that include depression, irritability, outbursts of temper, and apathy. Other personality changes may occur, such as the person becoming tactless or thoughtless. These problems often disrupt family life and practical ways have to be found to get around the difficulties caused. In this chapter I have focused on the carer. As the disease progresses the patient is less aware of the effects of their behaviour on others. In my experience, it is usually the carer who complains about the behavioural and emotional problems.

When do these problems occur?

Changes in mood or behaviour may occur before the start of clear-cut neurological signs. The changes may cause difficulties at work or in maintaining the usual household chores. If mood and behaviour changes coincide with neurological signs of Huntington's disease or occur after they are present, then it is not difficult to say that they are related to the condition. On the other hand, if they occur before neurological signs have become evident, then your doctor will have to keep an open mind as to whether or not Huntington's disease has started.

Problem behaviours

It may be helpful to take these problems in turn, realizing that some may be more prominent than others in any particular individual with Huntington's disease. There are no specific treatments for these behaviours, but I will describe some drugs that may be helpful at the end of the chapter.

Becoming less perceptive

One common feature of Huntington's disease is a lack of perception; you may find that your partner becomes focused on themselves and their needs, and is less perceptive to your needs. An example might be that he or she wants something and does not appreciate or perceive that you are tired and that it would be reasonable to wait.

Depression

Depression is a common human response to a variety of situations, and given a particular situation or loss, it might be very understandable that a person becomes depressed. Depression is a common feature of Huntington's disease; in some studies it is present in approximately a third of cases. The level of depression needs to be assessed in the context of the other problems that are described. Most of us can relate to the idea of feeling sad or down, becoming tearful, and not enjoying activities. It is important to have an idea about how often these problems occur; for example, once a week, several times a week or almost every day. A question that a doctor might ask is whether the depression or sadness responds to the person being cheered up or whether it has an adverse effect on normal daily activities.

Although there is no treatment for Huntington's disease as such, it is important to emphasize that some of the features, particularly depression and irritability, are treated using drugs that are currently available.

Apathy

The changes in the brain may result in apathy. You may find that your relative does not initiate conversations or activities and needs to be encouraged to do things that were routine a little while ago. They may, however, respond to gentle prompting. If the apathy is more pronounced, the person may take considerable persuasion to do tasks: he or she may be content to sit and watch a succession of television programmes or DVDs. A person can have a loss of interest without being depressed; however, it may be difficult to tell the difference between the two. If there is doubt, it may be better to provide antidepressant medication.

Irritability

We all have an idea about what being irritable means. Again, irritability is a normal human response. If any of us are a little tired and/or a little hungry and trying to focus on doing two things at the same time (or more accurately, switch between tasks) and someone comes and asks us a question, which in other circumstances may be trivial, then the response may well be irritation. I am sure you have come across this at home or at work. The problem with Huntington's disease is that the threshold may be set much lower, so that the irritability is both more frequent and occurs over more trivial issues. The irritability, and subsequent aggression, may be one of the more difficult aspects of Huntington's disease for the family. If the irritability is troublesome then a practical solution is for you, the relative or carer, to try to assess what triggers the irritability and avoid those triggers. This brings up a general point: the person with Huntington's disease has difficulty changing his or her behaviour, so you may have to consider what modifications you can make to your behaviour to avoid a confrontation.

Aggression

A consequence of irritability and frustration is that the person for whom you are caring may become aggressive. The aggression may take the form of verbal outbursts that do not cause much of a problem for the other members of the household, or the person may become abusive, hit the furniture or slam doors. Obviously, if aggression is severe it can result in actual physical violence. Apart from practical solutions of avoiding confrontations, it is important to seek medical help with drugs if aggression starts to become a problem.

Appearance

Someone with Huntington's disease may well lose pride in their personal appearance, which can lead to problems with washing, dressing, and shaving. Part of the problem may be related to apathy and part of the problem may be a depressed mood. It is difficult to give specific advice on this except to try to encourage a routine without precipitating an outburst of temper. Again, telling someone with Huntington's disease to wash and dress is unlikely to work; although it can be more difficult, it is better to try gentle persuasion. If someone with Huntington's disease is living largely on their own, these problems may easily result in an unkempt appearance.

Preoccupations

Being preoccupied with a particular topic, such as asking for the same thing over and over again, constantly coming back to the same topic, or insisting on doing something that is clearly not going to work, may be another source of difficulty. Again, this can happen to any of us, but it may be significant enough to cause problems for other family members or carers. The only solution is to try to accept that the behaviour is not going to change and to alter your own response.

ⓘ Patient's perspective

I am grateful to the family member who sent me this quote; he wishes to remain anonymous. The first part, about the dishwasher tablets, illustrates the need to accept that his partner is not going to change, so the only solution is for him to change. He has expressed very well the point that it is often essential to learn to anticipate problems and avoid minor issues becoming a serious problem. I have also often come across the problem of someone agreeing to go out and then changing their mind at the last minute. With experience this too can be anticipated and others forewarned that this may happen.

"While my wife finishes breakfast and starts the ritual of tidying the kitchen and loading the dishwasher, an increasingly obsessive act that will take two-plus hours, I sort through the bins for the financial papers tidied away yesterday and then take the rest of the family out to the shops.

Thirty minutes later when we get back we are in crisis and on the verge of a tantrum—we are about to run out of dishwasher tablets. Despite having literally a year's supply in the cupboard we know from bitter past experience that having reached this tipping point the only way to resolve this situation before anything else is to go back out and get six new boxes. Once an idea takes root, rational discussion is not an option and anything other than hard evidence that the problem is solved will only escalate the situation. It's not always possible to give the hard evidence so it's better to try to anticipate events, establish routines, and create a framework to minimize the scope for wholly disproportionate responses to fairly minor items.

This behaviour can be a bit of a shocker for visitors and is wearing for all.

We are going out this afternoon to a social gathering—a friend's children's christening—so to speed things up my wife agrees to let me help her shower but not dress. However it's now 11.30 and time for a high-calorie snack. She needs about 5,000 kcal/day to keep her weight stable.

The shower and hairwash is a success and we have plenty of time to dress and get round to our friends for 2.30. At 2.00 as we need to leave my wife declares she doesn't want to go and that I should go by myself but leave the children. Debate is fruitless. This is a unilateral decision of the type that makes coping and deciding as a couple difficult."

Anxiety

As with the other behaviours that can be a problem, this is a normal human response. We might all feel a little anxious if we have to go somewhere new but the anxiety is usually controlled. The issue is that a person with Huntington's disease may become anxious and tense more easily. This may manifest itself as pacing up and down, or being much more worried than could be expected in a given situation. If it is a significant problem, the person may want to avoid the situation and decide not to go out.

Can we explain the irritability and apathy further?

The brain has sometimes been likened to a computer. In many ways it is better than a computer because it can plan ahead, can switch between several tasks, and can cope with new information to change a plan. A simple example of switching between tasks would be preparing a meal whilst talking to the children about their activities at school. Similar situations occur at work, where it is possible to be doing a task whilst continuing a conversation with a colleague. Planning ahead is all very well, but it is frequently the case that during the day something occurs and new plans have to be made. These aspects of brain activity can be described as **executive functions** (e.g., planning ahead) and **cognitive flexibility** (being able to concentrate on more than one task and to adapt your plans in the light of new information). It is these functions that are impaired in Huntington's disease. It may now be easier to understand why someone with Huntington's disease loses drive and initiative and in consequence appears apathetic. Similarly, the patient can become overloaded with tasks or have difficulty adapting to changing situations and respond with what seems to be unreasonable irritability and outbursts of temper.

Trying to solve the problem is more difficult than describing it. A direct confrontation is unlikely to help, so other strategies have to be devised, such as avoiding precipitating factors, avoiding the need to concentrate on several tasks at once, having some structure to the day, and encouraging the person to participate in joint activities for as long as possible. In general terms it is better to try these methods rather than immediately turning to drugs. Some of these problems can be explained by changes that occur in the brain. These are discussed again in Chapter 9.

Sleep

Altered sleep patterns, which result in someone with Huntington's disease being restless at night, can be very disruptive of family life. Sleep disturbance may be a clue to the fact that someone is depressed. If this is the case then treating the depression may help. An alternative explanation is that a person with Huntington's disease may spend parts of the day dozing and, as a result, may be restless during the night when the rest of the family are trying to sleep. If apathy and constant cat-naps during the day are a problem then it may be possible to encourage some additional participation in household activities.

Memory

In Huntington's disease, the memory does become impaired but it is not completely lost. It may be that going shopping is more difficult because organizing the items to be remembered is a problem, so making a list is clearly important. Obviously, as the disease progresses the problem worsens. One difference between patients with Huntington's disease and Alzheimer's disease can be demonstrated with a test. Both groups of patients may have difficulty learning a list of unrelated words. However, someone with Huntington's disease will respond to cues, such as being told about an image that links the words together. This strategy does not work for someone with Alzheimer's disease, and their score on the test will be much the same whether or not cues are used.

Cognitive impairment

Although the term **dementia** is medically correct, I have decided not to use this as a paragraph heading. This may seem surprising, since the word 'dementia' is easier to understand than the alternative of 'cognitive impairment'. This obviously reflects my own preference, but I want to stress that the problems seen in people with Huntington's disease are different from the more global difficulties seen in people with Alzheimer's disease. We should not assume that a person with Huntington's disease has lost the ability to comprehend what is being said because of their appearance and speech difficulties. I want to return to this theme on page 103 when considering some of the changes that take place in the brain.

Sexual problems

It is difficult to know the extent of sexual problems in families. In my experience with patients, loss of sex drive is extremely common; however, this is not the impression that is given in some medical articles.

Some years ago doctors published case reports and described the worst cases they had seen. This is understandable, in the sense that we all remember unusual or striking cases. The problem with this approach is that it does not give a clear picture of what is happening in Huntington's disease families in general as compared to families without Huntington's disease. We can note that in his original paper, George Huntington described two married men with the disease whose wives were living, who were constantly making love to some young lady or other. The point I want to make is that, as we all know, this behaviour may equally well be seen in men who do not have Huntington's disease.

Although loss of sex drive is usual, this is not always the case. A person with Huntington's disease may lose some of the social inhibitions that normally govern behaviour. This process is called **disinhibition**. We have all seen or experienced disinhibited behaviour associated with drinking too much alcohol. The result of disinhibition for someone with Huntington's disease can be sexual behaviour or remarks that are inappropriate at a particular time or place. This can be embarrassing to other members of the family, who may find it difficult to understand and control.

A person with Huntington's disease may think he or she is less attractive and need reassurance. Occasionally, someone can falsely believe that their partner is having an affair. This is called **morbid jealousy**. If this occurs, then you may not be able to solve the problem by reassurance and may have to seek help, initially from your family doctor and then perhaps from a hospital clinic.

Which psychiatric illnesses occur in Huntington's disease?

The answer to this question is 'almost any'. However, among the various psychiatric illnesses that occur in Huntington's disease, depression is the most common. In most surveys of Huntington's disease, depression is the most frequent psychiatric diagnosis. Unlike the movement disorder, this problem needs to be recognized and treated with medication. Whilst the movement disorder may be obvious to your doctor, signs of a depressed mood have to be sought actively. Someone with Huntington's disease may find it difficult to describe their feelings, but could well admit to lack of self-esteem, feeling miserable, having difficulty with sleeping, and a general loss of appetite and interest in their usual activities.

Some people with severe depression can have false beliefs or **delusions**. One delusion was mentioned earlier in relation to morbid jealousy. Unlike in schizophrenia, these delusions can be understood in terms of the person's depressed mood and feelings of unworthiness. A doctor may check for paranoia by asking if the person thinks they are being watched or that people are talking about them. Another question may relate to whether the person believes that they are receiving messages from the television.

When we think of mood changes we most commonly think of depression, but of course the opposite mood swing is **mania**. This means that the person is extremely active and rushes about undertaking a lot of projects in a very pressured way. If this happens, then some very poor decisions can be made and a lot of money spent inadvisably. Although not common, this can occur in Huntington's disease.

Another well-known psychiatric problem is **hallucinations**. A doctor checking to make sure these are not present may ask if the person hears voices that other people do not hear or whether they have visions that other people cannot see.

Leaving aside depression, only a small percentage of people with Huntington's disease develop these other, more severe psychiatric problems.

Is suicide associated with Huntington's disease?

Many studies have shown an increased rate of suicide in the families with Huntington's disease compared with non-Huntington's disease families. Although suicides do occur, they are still rare events. In general terms, if someone with Huntington's disease is going to commit suicide then it is most likely to occur in the early stages of the disease. We need to be careful in distinguishing between someone who says that if things get bad in the future they would think about suicide but has really no specific plan, and someone who is actively planning an event or who has attempted suicide in the past.

Is alcohol a problem?

Many people with Huntington's disease find that a modest amount of alcohol has a more significant effect on them than previously. Indeed, people often complain that neighbours mistakenly accuse them of being drunk because of the movement disorder.

Drinking excess alcohol will cause problems whether or not you have Huntington's disease. As problems with alcohol occur in the general population, so they also occur in people with Huntington's disease. As may be expected, if someone has a drink problem in addition to Huntington's disease then the behaviour problems are much worsened.

Medication for psychiatric and behavioural problems

In the last chapter I stressed the need to avoid immediately turning to drugs to treat the movement disorder. In this chapter I want to indicate that, although non-drug treatments should be tried first, psychiatric symptoms may well need to be treated with drugs. A side effect of some of the treatments for psychiatric disorders is that they also slow down some of the choreic movements. I have decided not to give a list of the various types of drugs that are available, in part because no one particular drug has been shown to be more useful than another. Many professionals feel strongly that the problems associated with depression and irritability need to be treated with drugs. This means that many patients are prescribed an antidepressant. Treatment of the irritability may involve use of drugs that block the chemical dopamine in the brain. This is the same class of drug that may be used to treat the movement disorder. An alternative group of drugs for treating irritability is called beta-blockers. Until specific treatments become available that alter the damage to the nerve cells, we rely on treating the symptoms. Consequently, many patients may end up on a combination of a drug that blocks or depletes dopamine and an antidepressant.

➡ Summary

♦ Changes in personality and behaviour occur early in the course of the disease and can be present before the neurological problems begin.

♦ It is difficult to describe the full range of behaviour, but apathy, irritability, and outbursts of temper are common problems.

♦ A wide range of psychiatric problems occur in Huntington's disease, of which depression is common and needs to be treated. These frequently cause more problems for the patient's family than the movement disorder.

♦ There is no psychiatric illness or behaviour pattern that affects only people with Huntington's disease. The same problems can occur in people who do not have the gene for Huntington's disease.

4

Juvenile Huntington's disease

> ### ➡ Key points
>
> ◆ Juvenile Huntington's disease is not a separate condition, but there are some aspects that differ from the more typical adult onset.
>
> ◆ The definition is onset of the condition under the age of 20 years.
>
> ◆ Approximately 5 per cent of those with Huntington's disease meet this definition.
>
> ◆ Very early onset in childhood is rare but can happen.

The phrase 'juvenile Huntington's disease' or JHD is potentially alarming, as it implies children can develop the condition. An inspection of the graph showing age at onset (see Fig. 1.2 in Chapter 1) shows that, although it is uncommon, onset can occur at a young age.

The definition of JHD is onset under the age of 20 years. In one sense, the choice of 20 years is arbitrary, although it is convenient as it allows doctors to distinguish those rare cases with an onset under the age of 10 years and those with an onset between 10 and 20 years. There is going to be very little difference in the clinical features of someone with an age at onset of 19 years versus 21 or 22 years. One consequence of the definition is that if someone is now 29 or 30 years old but had onset when they were less than 20 years old, they will still be classed as JHD.

Why use the term JHD?

In the chapters on the clinical features, I hoped to convey the sense that within the pattern of Huntington's disease there is still variation. Typically, chorea starts early, but as time goes by individuals may develop slowness of movement and even unusual postures of the limbs (called dystonia). When Huntington's disease develops at an early age, the slowness of movement and unusual postures may be more prominent and the chorea less marked. During the twentieth century, doctors used various terms to describe the pattern of features when chorea is not a prominent feature. Using some of these terms may add to confusion but, given that this pattern is more frequently associated with a young age at onset, the term 'juvenile Huntington's disease' is helpful. Juvenile Huntington's disease is not a separate condition, but rather a useful way of describing features that are at one end of the spectrum of features seen with Huntington's disease. The term may also be helpful because it recognizes that Huntington's disease is happening at a very different time in the person's life. For example, a young person may be at school, developing friendships and independence.

How frequent is JHD?

It is difficult to estimate how frequent JHD is. When researchers estimate the number of cases of Huntington's disease in a population, they often include a brief summary of the number of cases with an onset age of less than 20 years. The results from surveys vary, but an approximate estimate is 5 per cent. This figure requires a little more explanation. If, in round figures, 10 people in 100,000 have HD, then in a country with a population of 60 million at any given time there will be approximately 6,000 people affected with HD. If 5 per cent of these have an onset age of less than 20 years then there should be approximately 300 cases. This looks like a lot of cases, and is probably more than most doctors would think would be the case, based on their clinical experience. The term JHD invites us to think of children, but of course the definition includes those individuals currently in their twenties or possibly thirties who started having JHD when they were teenagers. Most doctors, even those with a special interest in HD, will not have much experience of managing children and young people with HD.

What are the clinical features of JHD?

As with HD in general, it is easier to describe the motor features than other clinical features. Children and young people tend to have problems with slowness of movement and clumsiness. There is often difficulty with speech.

One problem is that the muscles contract more than they should, so there can be problems with abnormal posture of the limbs. One of the problems can be muscle cramps, which may be painful. The muscles may contract and relax quickly, which gives a jerky movement that doctors describe as **myoclonus** or myoclonic jerks. Chorea may occur in younger people with Huntington's disease, but it is much less prominent than the general slowness of movement. Epilepsy may occur in HD, but it is more common in the juvenile form.

Behavioural problems occur in JHD just as much as in the more typical form, but this may be more difficult to explain or understand. If a child or young person becomes difficult at home then the parent may become worried that this is the start of HD, particularly as the family may have direct experience of HD themselves. The problems with behaviour are likely to occur before the onset of clear-cut problems with movement. This poses particular problems for diagnosis. Another feature of JHD is a decline in school performance, which can result in difficulties until the diagnosis is made.

ⓘ Patient's perspective

This quote illustrates that a parent or guardian may well be aware of subtle changes long before anyone else.

"When she was thirteen, I started to notice very, very, very, very small changes, so small nobody else could see them, and I kept looking and I couldn't even describe what those changes were, they were so minute. At one point, after a few months obviously, they were a bit more noticeable, but again other people still didn't notice. Other close family members couldn't see anything different in her."

Challenges for diagnosis: frustration for parents

Parents, including foster or adoptive parents, may realize that there are problems for a child or young person long before clinical signs related to movement are apparent to a doctor. In some cases, this has the potential to set up a conflict between the two over the use of the genetic test. Seen from the perspective of the parent, a diagnosis can help to explain problems and a definite diagnosis can result in access to other services such as additional help at school or support from social services. Not making a diagnosis results in continuing uncertainty and the possibility that the poor behaviour is being explained by others as the result of problems in the family and more specifically with parenting skills. As time goes by the parents may become more convinced that JHD is a reasonable and rational explanation for the problems and become increasingly frustrated by a doctor refusing to use the genetic test. Equally, there may be some parents who will be very nervous about receiving the diagnosis, as it may give them the definite answer that the problems are caused by Huntington's disease.

I now want to consider the same issue from the perspective of the doctors. Although it is possible to treat some of the symptoms of Huntington's disease, there is no treatment that will delay onset or reduce the underlying damage to the nerve cells in the brain. The gene for Huntington's disease is larger than normal, and this is described in much more detail in Chapter 6. If an individual has this larger gene, it will show up in a genetic test result, irrespective of when the test is done. In adults who have a 50 per cent risk of inheriting the condition, the genetic test is used cautiously. Care is taken to ensure that unaffected adults having a predictive test are not being coerced in any way and that their decision to have the test has been stable over a period of time. It is difficult to know how many people at risk of HD choose to be tested, but it is reasonable to assume that the majority choose not to have the test.

As far as children are concerned, genetic tests should be used for the benefit of the child or young person themself. If the onset of JHD is non-specific then the behavioural problems may not be due to HD. If the genetic test is done at this stage then a normal result rules out the diagnosis. If the result comes back showing a very large increase in size, as shown in Figure 6.1 (see Chapter 6), then it is likely that there will be juvenile onset. A problem arises if the result comes back with an abnormal but not very large size. In this circumstance it is not possible to say whether the problems are related to JHD; all that can be said is that the child or young person has inherited the gene. If the problems are unrelated to HD then a predictive test will have been done without consent. The consequence of this policy is that there is often a delay of some years in making a diagnosis, because doctors often wait until there are problems with movement before thinking that the child or young person is affected and then use the test to confirm their clinical diagnosis. The problem is that the genetic test says whether or not the abnormal gene is present, but deciding when the condition has started is still a matter of doctors recognizing a pattern of features in a patient and making a clinical judgement.

📄 Case study

This anecdote, from a colleague, illustrates the reason for caution. Unfortunately, there is not a lot of detail about such cases, where children have been tested in good faith and the test result was abnormal but not very large (with repeats numbering in the low or mid-forties; see Chapter 6).

A young person was tested in childhood because the family and doctors felt HD was starting. This was not the case but the result was just over 40 repeats. That individual is now well as a young adult. They are coping well but would have preferred not to have had a predictive test.

Given these two perspectives and the fact that most doctors have not seen many young people with HD, what can be done to improve the current situation? My suggestions would be for the concerns of the parent or guardian to be taken seriously, whilst explaining the need for caution. Basing a diagnosis on behavioural problems is difficult but it may help to ask a psychologist working for the education department to formally assess and document whether there has been a decline in school performance. In time, other tests may be developed that will distinguish between people in the pre-symptomatic stage of the condition and those who are affected. This point is explored again in Chapter 11. Although this explanation may not solve the frustration some families have experienced, it may go some way towards explaining it.

Genetic aspects of JHD

I will discuss the issue of the enlarged gene in detail in Chapter 6. In general terms, the larger the gene, the earlier the average age of onset. I want to emphasize that this is an average, because a group of individuals with the same sized gene can still have a wide range of age of onset. We would expect individuals with a young age of onset to have the largest genes. This is true to an extent but there is not an absolute cut-off that distinguishes an age of onset of less than 20 years.

Before the gene was identified, it was recognized that more people with JHD had an affected father than an affected mother. Again, this is on average, but it can now be explained that large increases in the size of the HD gene are more likely to occur in sperm than in egg cells. It is worth emphasizing again that JHD is rare and that most parents do not have children with JHD. Also, it is not the case that most fathers who pass on the gene to their child find that the child develops JHD. I will come back to the genetic aspects of JHD in Chapter 6.

Management issues for JHD

As with HD in general, there are no specific recommendations for treating children and young people with JHD. The aims are to relieve symptoms but as the motor symptoms are more to do with muscle stiffness a different range of drugs are used, compared with the more typical adult form. Given that there are no specific recommendations, I hesitate to name particular drugs; it is more important to have a treatment that is effective for the individual child or young person. In general terms, we can say that in the typical form of HD it is common to use drugs that block the effects of a chemical in the brain called dopamine. It may be that in JHD symptoms can be relieved by doing the opposite; that is stimulating dopamine. A drug that helps with muscle spasms is called baclofen, and this may also be used. Other drugs are helpful to control mood and epilepsy.

As with the more typical form of Huntington's disease, the behavioural problems may be more difficult to understand and manage than the physical problems.

> ### ⓘ Patient's perspective
>
> "The mobility problems aren't as bad but it's all these temper outbursts and lack of reasoning, behavioural problems, which are a lot harder to cope with than looking after [his father] who's not terribly mobile."

Why study JHD?

Juvenile Huntington's disease is rare, so most doctors do not have a great deal of experience in managing the condition. In order to improve treatments we need to understand what treatments are currently being prescribed. We also need to develop methods of assessing children and young people to compare different treatments so that it is possible to make recommendations. Given that this is a rare form of HD, we need to establish studies that involve doctors in different countries. This form of network research is being developed and is described in Chapter 11. One interesting point is that no animal apart from humans develops HD. When the gene was cloned, scientists were able to introduce the abnormal gene into laboratory animals. Interestingly, especially large forms of the abnormal gene were used in this research, so in fact the disease in these laboratory animals more closely resembles the juvenile form of HD than the adult form.

5

The genetics of Huntington's disease

> ## ➲ Key points
>
> ◆ We have two copies of all our genetic material.
>
> ◆ Individual genes cannot be seen with a microscope but are packaged into structures called chromosomes.
>
> ◆ Huntington's disease results from a mistake in one copy of a gene on chromosome 4.
>
> ◆ The effect of the copy with the mistake dominates over the normal copy.
>
> ◆ If someone has Huntington's disease, then on average half their children will inherit the condition.
>
> ◆ The mistake is an enlargement in the first part of the gene.
>
> ◆ Genes make proteins. The Huntington's gene make a protein called huntingtin. This protein is larger than it should be and causes problems for some cells in the brain.

Common errors, misunderstandings, and myths

Despite the increase in genetic services and greater awareness of Huntington's disease in the media over the last ten to twenty years, I still meet families where the comments in the box below are made. I can understand how this may happen. Individuals will look at the pattern in their own family and come to a conclusion that seems to explain what has happened. The problem with this approach is that the pattern is based on a few individuals and at most can cover information from only three generations. I am taking a risk in mentioning incorrect information; I would not want someone to miss the important point that this chapter is about explaining why this information is incorrect.

> ## ⊗ Myths about Huntington's disease
>
> Huntington's disease only (or mostly) affects boys.
>
> Huntington's disease only (or mostly) affects girls.
>
> Huntington's disease always misses the first child (or some other pattern).
>
> Huntington's disease can skip a generation.

Why do we have genes?

It may be useful to remember that your body is composed of millions of cells, and that these cells have specialist functions. Each cell contains a full complement of genetic material. The genes are the instructions for a cell to make proteins. Some proteins are present in every cell, whereas other proteins are only present in particular cell types. The proteins present in a liver cell will be different from those present in a muscle cell, and different again from those in a nerve cell of the brain. The different proteins allow the cell to grow and have specialized functions. Put very simply, a gene is the code for a particular protein. We could ask if different cells contain different genes, but the answer to this is no. Each cell has two copies of every gene so it follows that in any particular cell a lot of genes are inactive.

Can we see individual genes?

No, we cannot see the individual genes under a microscope. Most people are familiar with the idea that the genetic code is in the DNA molecule. DNA is a long molecule and has the structure of a double helix. In a cell, the DNA is found in a part of the cell called the nucleus. As a cell divides, the DNA molecule gets wound up to form a structure called a chromosome, as shown in Figure 5.1. We have two copies of all our genetic material: half comes from the mother and half comes from the father, and therefore the chromosomes are in pairs. Since each cell contains a full copy of the genetic material it is possible to grow some cells from a blood sample in the laboratory and know that the chromosomes in these cells look the same as those present in other body cells. The chromosomes shown in Figure 5.1 came from one cell of a male individual. Essentially, dividing cells were put under a microscope and the chromosomes were stained to give a specific striped pattern. This was examined under the microscope and a digital image was taken. The chromosomes were then lined up in their pairs and the image recorded. It is clear that each cell has 46 chromosomes and that they are in 23 pairs. The chromosomes in the first 22 pairs are equal and these are called the **autosomes**. The last pair of chromosomes in this cell are unequal; they are the **X** and **Y** chromosomes, which indicates that this cell came from a male. A cell from a female would have two X chromosomes. The last pair of chromosomes are called the **sex chromosomes**, but they do not feature in the story of Huntington's disease.

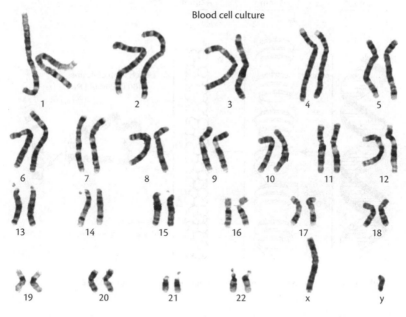

Blood cell culture

46,XY Normal male karyotype

Figure 5.1 Photograph of the chromosomes from a single cell. The chromosomes are in pairs and are arranged in order of size. The last pair are called the sex chromosomes. In this case there is an X and a Y, so the cell came from a male. Photograph courtesy of Mr M. Dyson.

The idea that the genetic material is contained within the chromosomes was known in the first half of the twentieth century, but correctly counting that human cells had 46 chromosomes in 23 pairs did not occur until 1956. It is interesting to think that genetics has come a very long way in just over fifty years.

If we cannot see the individual genes, where are they on the chromosome? The answer is that a chromosome consists of a DNA molecule that is coiled up very tightly. Figure 5.2 shows a tiny section of a chromosome in which a tiny part of the DNA molecule is unwound. A gene is a section of the DNA molecule that contains the message to make a particular protein.

A major scientific task was to find out which genes were on which chromosome. A few genes were mapped to specific chromosomes, but it was not until the 1980s that mapping genes to specific chromosomes gathered momentum.

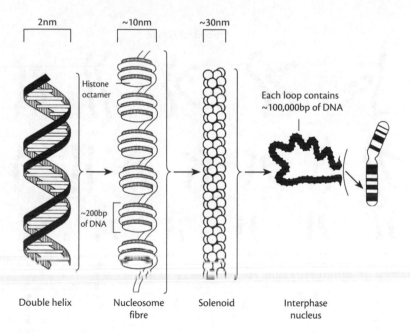

Figure 5.2 Diagram to show the relationship between DNA and a chromosome. The DNA molecule is wound onto proteins called histones. Coiling the DNA in this way is like putting it around cotton reels. The DNA can be coiled again and again until the chromosome structure has been achieved. A gene is a stretch of the DNA molecule. Although it is possible to see a chromosome under the microscope, it is impossible to see the individual genes this way. bp = base pairs.

As noted in Chapter 1, the gene for Huntington's disease was mapped to the tip of chromosome 4 in 1983 and the precise location was identified in 1993.

How does a gene code for a protein

The DNA molecule consists of two strings of chemicals, which are usually called by the letters 'A', 'C', 'G', and 'T' after the first letters of their chemical names: 'A' for adenine, 'C' for cytosine, 'G' for guanine, and 'T' for thymine. A very tiny section of the DNA molecule can be represented by these letters, as shown in Figure 5.3. A DNA molecule can always copy itself because A always pairs with T, and C always pairs with G. Most of the DNA molecule does not code for anything, but, at particular points, sections of the DNA molecule code for the building blocks of protein. Sections of the DNA molecule which code for proteins are called genes. Within a gene, a group of three letters, say 'CAG', codes for one of the building blocks of a protein; another group of three letters, say 'GAA', codes for a different building block of a protein. A group of three letters which codes for a protein building block is called a **triplet**.

What about eggs and sperm?

It is common knowledge that we have two copies of our genes and that we inherit half our genes from our mother and half from our father. It is easy to see that when an egg is made (before it is fertilized) it contains one copy of chromosome 1, one of chromosome 2, one of chromosome 3, etc., and, since eggs are made by females, one X chromosome. Similarly, a sperm contains

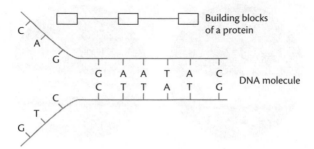

Figure 5.3 Diagram to show the four-letter code of the DNA molecule. The DNA molecule consists of a double helix. There are rules for the way the letters are arranged. 'A' always pairs with 'T' and 'C' pairs with 'G'. In a stretch of DNA which is a gene, three letters code for one of the building blocks of a protein.

one chromosome 1, one chromosome 2, one chromosome 3, etc., and, since sperm are made by males, it will contain either an X chromosome or a Y chromosome. In this way, when an egg and sperm fuse, the new cell or future child has two copies of each gene, one from the father and one from the mother. If the sperm contained an X chromosome, the future child will be a girl, and if it contained a Y chromosome, the future child will be a boy (see Fig. 5.4). (This is a point that was lost on King Henry VIII.)

The gene for Huntington's disease is located on chromosome 4. Therefore, the condition can affect both males and females. This means that 50 per cent of the cases of Huntington's disease are male and 50 per cent are female (see

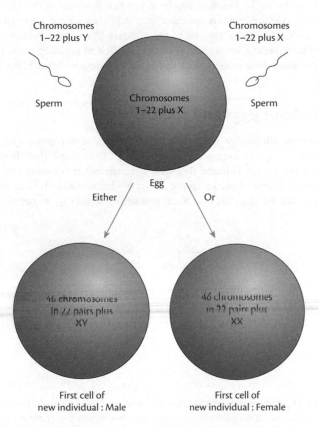

Figure 5.4 Diagram to show that the sex of a baby is determined by the sperm (see text for an explanation).

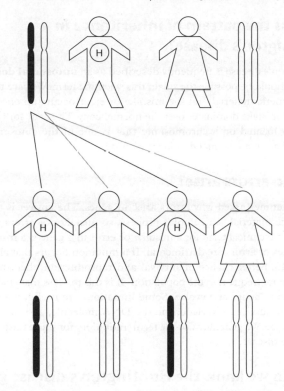

Figure 5.5 Diagram to show the pattern of inheritance of Huntington's disease. In this diagram the father has the Huntington's disease gene; he has one chromosome 4 with the Huntington's disease gene and one normal chromosome 4. Each parent gives a chromosome 4 to the children. The children are bound to get a normal chromosome 4 from the mother but it is 50:50 whether they get the chromosome 4 with Huntington's disease or the normal one from the father. It makes no difference whether the children are boys or girls.

The diagram could be redrawn with the mother having the Huntington's disease gene and the father unaffected. The effect for the children would be exactly the same; the chance of them inheriting the Huntington's disease gene would still be 50:50 and it would make no difference whether they were boys or girls.

Fig. 5.5). Usually we only know a few members of our immediate family. It may the case that, by chance, in your family more males than females are affected, or the other way around, but if we add up information from a lot of families then the pattern of equal proportions of males and females being affected will emerge.

What is the pattern of inheritance in Huntington's disease?

Huntington's disease is frequently described as an **autosomal dominant** disorder. It should be possible to explain this scientific term. We have two copies of all our genetic material, but the mistake or error occurs on one copy of the gene. The mistake dominates over the normal copy. The gene for Huntington's disease is located on a chromosome that is one of the autosomes, so it is described as an autosomal dominant disorder.

Why do errors arise?

I am sometimes asked why errors arise in genes. The answer is that copying the genetic material is a complex process, so mistakes or errors occasionally occur. The technical term for a mistake or error in a gene is a **mutation**. Not all mistakes or errors are detrimental. If a mutation occurs that allows a plant or animal a better chance of survival and reproduction, then that gene will become more frequent in the population. It is this process that enables animals and plants to adapt and evolve. Some mutations are useful, the majority are neutral and just cause variations in the DNA molecule, and some, of course, cause disease. We generally use the term 'mutation' for those mistakes in genes that cause disease.

How do we know the Huntington's disease gene is on chromosome 4?

I have included this section for interest, but, as it is a potted history of the discovery of the gene, it can be skipped. The story starts back in the nineteenth century with Gregor Mendel and his peas. Gregor Mendel was an Austrian monk who worked out some laws of genetic inheritance from his work growing different varieties of peas in his monastery garden. He discovered that one copy of each gene pair is transmitted during reproduction, and that the different gene pairs are inherited independently of one another. Most of this is correct, but of course Mendel was not aware that genes are packaged on chromosomes. When eggs and sperm are forming, an interesting thing happens to the chromosomes, as shown in Figure 5.6. The chromosomes line up in their pairs and exchange genetic material. If gene pairs are far apart on the same chromosome, or are on completely separate chromosomes, then they will be inherited independently, just as Mendel predicted. However, if they are close together on the same chromosome, then it is less likely that they will be separated by

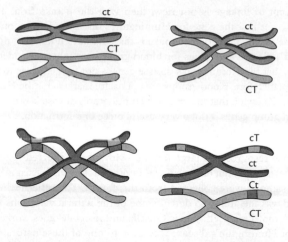

Figure 5.6 Diagram to show how genetic material is exchanged between chromosomes before eggs and sperm are formed. In this diagram the letters **c**, **C**, **t**, and **T** represent different forms of two genes. Before eggs and sperm form, the chromosome pairs duplicate but do not completely separate (top left). They then come together in their pairs (top right). Genetic material is exchanged between the chromosome pairs (bottom left). Then the chromosomes separate (bottom right). In this way the genetic material on the chromosome pairs is shuffled and one of the resulting chromosomes goes into either the egg or the sperm.

a crossover, in which case they will be inherited together far more often than we would expect. The technical term for gene pairs being close together on the same chromosome is **linkage**. The concept of linkage is not new; it was described in the early years of the twentieth century. Linkage was first described in humans in 1937 by two British geneticists, Julia Bell and J. B. S. Haldane. They described the fact that the genes for haemophilia and colour-blindness were close together on the X chromosomes, but at the end of their paper they commented that it would be useful to find a marker (such as a gene for blood group) close to the Huntington's disease gene. In this context, a marker is a detectable genetic variation very close to the Huntington's disease gene. The marker has nothing to do with Huntington's disease other than being close to it on the chromosome. In the case of haemophilia and colour-blindness it is crucially important to realize that not all individuals with haemophilia are colour-blind, but rather that, if the two conditions occur together, they tend to stay together because the genes are next door to each other on the X chromosome.

If the concept of linkage is not new, then why did it take from 1937 until 1983 to discover that the gene for Huntington's disease is located on the tip of chromosome 4? The first point to make is that, in affected families, the gene for Huntington's disease and genes for blood groups are inherited independently. This means that the Huntington's disease gene is not located close to a gene for blood group; therefore, blood groups are not useful markers for the Huntington's disease gene. Knowing that the gene for Huntington's disease is not close to one of the blood group genes is not a very useful piece of information.

In order to locate the gene, several resources and techniques needed to come together. One resource was large families with lots of affected relatives alive. Such families are rare, but one very large family was known to exist in Venezuela, and blood samples were collected from this family. The other technique that was needed was the ability to detect some of the natural variations that occur in the DNA molecule itself. James Gusella and his colleagues worked to see if the gene for Huntington's disease was close to one of these natural variations in the DNA molecule in the Venezuelan family and one other large family. They were successful in identifying that the gene for Huntington's disease was close to one of these variations, and since the particular variation was at the tip of chromosome 4, it followed that the gene for Huntington's disease was also located at the same place.

This work was published in November 1983 and sparked a whole new line of enquiry. The first step was to discover if the gene for Huntington's disease was on chromosome 4 in all families. Several researchers, from different countries, tested families they were studying and concluded that yes, the mutation (or error) was on chromosome 4 in all families. This work took approximately two years, from 1984 to 1986. It was immediately realized that if the marker could be followed in a particular family, then unaffected offspring could be told whether or not they would develop Huntington's disease, depending on which form of the marker they had inherited (see Fig. 5.7). The issue of predictive testing is considered in more detail in the next chapter. For the moment, it is enough to say that guidelines were developed at this time so that predictive testing was introduced in a carefully considered and controlled way.

Predictive tests based on linkage studies were used from 1986 until 1993. Linkage-based tests are used occasionally for the special case of someone who wants a test in pregnancy, or on an embryo, but does not want to know whether they themselves have inherited the gene. I will come back to this form of testing in Chapter 8. However, the actual mutation in the gene was identified in 1993 and in general this has replaced the older test.

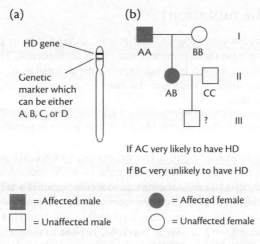

If AC very likely to have HD

If BC very unlikely to have HD

Figure 5.7 Diagram showing a predictive test using linkage. This takes advantage of the fact that a marker (or natural variation in the DNA molecule) was found that was very close to the Huntington's disease gene (a). The genetic marker occurs in several forms. In any one individual the form of the genetic marker next to the Huntington's disease gene is very unlikely to be shuffled when eggs and sperm form. By following the marker through a family as in (b) a prediction can be made. The mother in generation II has inherited Huntington's disease and marker **A** from her father. Marker **A** is not present in her husband so a prediction can be made for her son. This type of test is cumbersome and relies on a family study.

Why did it take ten years to identify the gene?

It is easy to look back and wonder why it took so long to identify the gene. The technology to identify a gene improved over the ten-year period. The basic idea was that if one marker could be found that was close to the gene, then other markers from the same region might be even closer. As a chromosome is a length of DNA, it was very important to know if the gene was closer to the tip of the chromosome or was on the other side of the marker. It was soon realized that the gene was closer to the tip, but it was not until many more sections of DNA had been identified that the precise location of the gene was known. It was then a case of identifying the genes in a very tiny area to see if one contained a mutation. The mutation was eventually found in a gene called *IT15*. This is an odd name, but it represents the laboratory name for one of the fragments of DNA from the critical area of chromosome 4. Once the gene was identified it was possible to identify the protein for which it was coding. This protein had not been recognized before and was named **huntingtin**.

What is the mutation?

Genes are divided into sections, and it was realized that in patients with Huntington's disease the first section was larger than normal. The size of the normal gene varies a little, but Huntington's disease genes are always large. This can be explained by looking at the exact sequence of coding letters from the start of the gene.

The code for one of the building blocks of huntingtin is repeated a number of times in normal genes. This code is CAG. So normal DNA has the code: CAGCAGCAGCAGCAG (etc.). The number of times CAG is repeated on a normal gene varies, but it is frequently from 15 to 20 times. A section of the DNA molecule that has this structure is sometimes called a **triplet repeat**, the triplet in this case being CAG. Patients with Huntington's disease have a CAG repeat size of 36 or more. This knowledge is summarized by scientists describing Huntington's disease as a **triplet repeat disorder**, an **unstable CAG repeat disorder** or a **CAG repeat expansion disorder**. These terms seem mysterious but are ways of summarizing the fact that within the first part of the gene there is a section that is larger than normal.

The building block of the protein coded by CAG is **glutamine**, so it follows that the first part of the huntingtin protein contains glutamine repeated a number of times, as shown in Figure 5.8. As we have seen earlier, many terms in medicine and science are derived from the Greek and Latin languages. The Greek word for many is 'poly', so this part of the protein is sometimes called a **polyglutamine tract**.

In someone with Huntington's disease the number of CAG repeats is 36 or more. If there are 36 or more repeats then the abnormal huntingtin protein will have 36 or more glutamines. The abnormal huntingtin protein has an **expanded polyglutamine tract** (see Fig. 5.9).

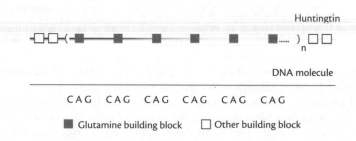

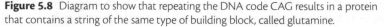

Figure 5.8 Diagram to show that repeating the DNA code CAG results in a protein that contains a string of the same type of building block, called glutamine.

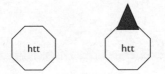

Figure 5.9 The normal-sized huntingtin protein (**htt**) has a particular shape, represented by the octagon. An abnormal huntingtin protein with the expanded polyglutamine repeat results in the protein represented by the addition of the triangle. Some of the effects of the abnormal protein are described further in Chapter 10.

It is now a relatively simple laboratory procedure to check the number of CAG repeats from a sample of a person's cells. For convenience, we most often use some cells from a blood sample. You have to remember that, apart from eggs and sperm, each cell has two copies of chromosome 4, so we get two results from each individual. If someone does not have Huntington's disease then both copies of the gene will contain CAG repeats in the normal size range. However, if someone has Huntington's disease, then one copy of the gene will be in the normal size range and the other copy will be in the Huntington's disease size range.

6

Laboratory testing

➜ Key points

◆ It is possible to measure the size of the first part of the gene for Huntington's disease so as to know how many CAG repeats are present in the gene.

◆ A gene with more than 36 repeats is abnormal but at this level the person may develop the disease late in life or even not at all.

◆ Above 40 repeats is definitely abnormal. A person with this result will definitely develop Huntington's disease.

◆ There is a trend for larger repeat sizes to be associated with an earlier age of onset but there is so much variation that it cannot help make a prediction for an individual.

Testing for Huntington's disease has now become a routine process for genetic laboratories. Although the technical aspects of the test have become more straightforward, interpreting the result can still raise issues and there are still important items to discuss during genetic counselling for someone who is at 50 per cent risk and who requests a predictive test. I will deal with the genetic counselling aspects of the Huntington's disease test in the next chapter.

How does the laboratory test work?

The essential step is to extract DNA from some cells. This is most conveniently done from a blood sample. There are laboratory techniques that allow a specific section of DNA to be amplified. In the case of testing for Huntington's disease, only the section that contains the CAG repeat is amplified. One of the chemicals used in the process is fluorescent so that the newly formed fragments of DNA can be recognized. As we have two copies of the gene, two different-sized fragments may be recognized. Clearly, if both copies of the gene have 18 repeats then only one size will be seen. Sizing of the fragments is now done using machines. The amplified DNA fragments are passed through a gel in a small tube called a capillary. A smaller fragment will travel faster than a larger fragment. As the fragments contain a fluorescent tag, they can be detected by a laser at the end of the capillary. If an individual has two genes with sizes of, say, 16 and 20 repeats, then both copies of the gene are in the normal size range and the person is unaffected. Similarly, if an individual is clearly affected with Huntington's disease then one gene should be in the normal size range and the other should be larger and in the abnormal size range. Results from some laboratory tests are shown in Figure 6.1.

Is there any overlap between the normal and Huntington's disease size ranges?

There may well be a small overlap. The upper end of the normal range may just overlap with the start of the Huntington's disease range. It is difficult to know about the upper end of the normal range in great detail because for the most part we only use the genetic test in the context of families where there is a concern about Huntington's disease. For the most part, genetic tests give a clear-cut answer, but the special case of results in the range of 36 to 39 repeats will be considered again in Chapter 8.

Is there any relationship between the size of the repeat and the age of onset of Huntington's disease?

The answer to this is 'yes'. In general terms, the larger the number of CAG repeats then the earlier the age of onset. This effect is shown in Figure 6.2. It was soon realized that, although there was a mathematical trend that worked for a large group of patients, it was not helpful for any particular individual. If you look carefully at Figure 6.2 you can see that for the common results of 40 to 60 repeats there is a very wide range of ages of onset. This means that, although the size of the CAG repeat has an important effect on the age of the onset, there must be other factors involved in determining the age of onset for a particular individual. For any individual patient, knowing the size of the CAG repeat does not help predict the age of onset.

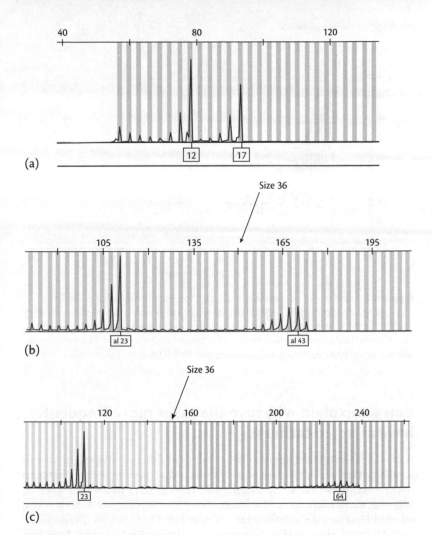

Figure 6.1 Results from three laboratory tests. Result (a) shows two normal-sized genes. This person is clearly unaffected. Result (b) shows a result with one normal-sized copy of the gene and one large-sized copy. This person has inherited the Huntington's disease gene. Result (c) comes from someone with a young age of onset. The laboratory technique amplifies the first part of the gene, which contains the repeated CAG sequence. The position of different-sized sections of DNA can be predicted; the position of a section with 36 repeats is indicated in (b) and (c). The size of the section of DNA can be counted from reference points (not shown). It is easier for shorter sections to be amplified, which explains why the peaks of the larger sections of DNA are smaller. Images courtesy of Dr J. Martindale.

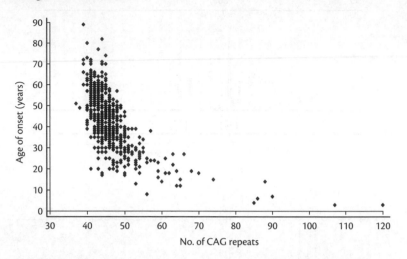

Figure 6.2 Number of CAG repeats versus age of onset. There is a clear trend for individuals with larger repeat sizes to have an earlier age of onset. However, if you look carefully at the individual repeat sizes you will see that there is a very large range in the age of onset. This means that we cannot tell when an individual with a particular repeat size will develop the condition. Image courtesy of Prof. F. Squitieri.

Can we explain why juvenile cases more frequently have affected fathers?

A case of juvenile Huntington's disease can have either an affected mother or an affected father. On the face of it, both should be equally likely. It has been noted since 1969 that in cases of juvenile Huntington's disease the affected parent is more likely to be the father. As we saw in Chapter 4, very young onset of Huntington's disease is rare. A man with Huntington's disease is not very likely to have a child with young-onset Huntington's disease. However, when it is the other way around, a person with young-onset disease is more likely to have an affected father than an affected mother.

It is now possible to explain this observation. If we consider a person with a normal number of repeats, say 17 repeats on one copy of the gene and 20 repeats on the other, then the vast majority of eggs or sperm will have either a gene with 17 repeats or 20 repeats. There may be the odd egg or sperm with 16 repeats or 18 repeats but these are very rare. On the whole, transmission of normal repeat sizes down the generations is reasonably stable (Fig. 6.3).

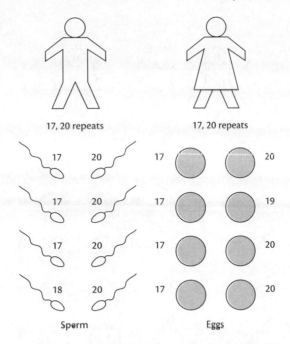

Figure 6.3 Diagram to show the stable inheritance of normal-sized CAG repeats in males and females. Only the odd egg or sperm contains a change from one of the original sizes.

By contrast, repeat sizes in the Huntington's disease range are *unstable* when transmitted down the generations. Although repeat sizes can increase or decrease in eggs and sperm, the general tendency is for them to become larger. The tendency for repeat sizes to increase is much greater in sperm than in eggs. This is shown in Figure 6.4. A man affected with Huntington's disease has basically two types of sperm: those with the normal-sized copy of the gene and those with the copy in the Huntington's disease size range. The sperm with the normal-sized copy of the gene will be as stable as before, but there will be considerable variation in the number of repeats in those sperm that contain the Huntington's disease gene. Very occasionally a sperm can form with a very large increase in the number of repeats. Although there is some variation of repeat size in eggs, such very large increases do not occur as frequently. Now that we know that differences occur in repeat sizes between eggs and sperm, it is easy to understand why more cases of juvenile onset have inherited their gene from their father.

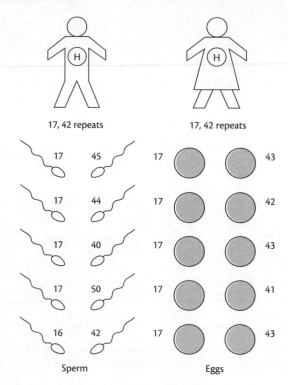

17, 42 repeats   17, 42 repeats

Sperm   Eggs

Figure 6.4 Diagram to show the unstable inheritance of CAG repeats in the Huntington's disease range. The Huntington's disease genes in the eggs and sperm are usually around the same size as in the parent, but in the case of a male an occasional sperm will have a very large increase in size.

Some scientists describe the nature of the Huntington's disease mutation by calling it an **unstable expansion of a trinucleotide repeat.** At first sight this seems very technical; however, given the explanations in the previous few sections, I hope you can see this is actually a neat summary of the mutation.

Can new mutations occur in Huntington's disease?

Before 1993 the answer to this question would probably have been 'not really'. It was long held that new mutations were exceptionally rare. It was not unknown for someone to have Huntington's disease and their parents to be unaffected, but this was often dismissed by saying there could have been non-paternity, or that one of the parents had died before they developed

Huntington's disease. However, now that we understand what is wrong with the gene, it has become easier to prove how new mutations arise.

Some people in the population have a normal gene with a repeat number in the high twenties and low thirties. As they have fewer than 36 repeats, they do not develop Huntington's disease. In the vast majority of cases the gene is transmitted to children without any increase in size, but just occasionally a man with this type of normal gene can produce a sperm that has a repeat size in the Huntington's disease range. If this happens then a new mutation has started. In some genetic disorders new mutations tend to arise more often in sperm, and Huntington's disease can be added to that list. If someone has a result in this size range then the chance of it expanding into the abnormal range is small, but it is disturbing because it is not quite a clear-cut normal result.

Does everyone with more than 36 repeats develop Huntington's disease?

In an earlier section I mentioned the occasional overlap between the size of normal genes and those that cause Huntington's disease, but there is also a second complication regarding the lower size limit of Huntington's disease genes.

Before the gene was identified, doctors were clear that if someone inherited the gene they would develop Huntington's disease, provided they lived long enough. The technical term for this is that Huntington's disease shows **full penetrance**. Not all genetic conditions show full penetrance. It is possible for someone to inherit a gene that causes a disease, to be unaffected themselves, and to pass the gene to a child who is then affected. When this happens the disease in question is described as showing **incomplete penetrance**.

If an individual has clear signs of Huntington's disease and a result between 36 and 39 repeats, then there is not a problem with interpreting the result, but if someone who is at 50 per cent risk has a test and one gene is in the normal range and the other is in the 36 to 39 range, then it is difficult to know whether or not that person will develop Huntington's disease late in life, or even not at all. One way of approaching this problem is to collect together information on the ages of onset of people with results in this size range. If this is done then it is possible to say that there is at least a 40 per cent chance the person will develop Huntington's disease after the age of 65 years and at least a 30 per cent chance they will develop the condition after the age of 75 years. There is a problem with this direct observational approach, because not every elderly unaffected person in the family will have been tested and their information will be missed from the study. Consequently, the actual chances of not being affected until later in life (or even not at all) may be higher than has been suggested. This is why I used the term 'at least'.

Summary of genetic test results

In 1998, a committee in North America published recommendations on how to report different types of results. This is summarized in Figure 6.5. Essentially, anything below 27 repeats is unequivocally normal. A result between 27 and 35 repeats is normal, but may expand in future generations. Between 36 and 39 repeats the result is abnormal, but there is the possibility of reduced penetrance. Above 40 repeats is unequivocally abnormal. A person at 50 per cent risk of developing Huntington's disease who has a predictive test result over 40 repeats will develop the condition, but it is not possible to say when the condition will start.

Information about juvenile Huntington's disease has been added to the diagram. Above 60 repeats is likely to be associated with onset under 20 years, but this is only an approximation. If you look carefully at Figure 6.2, you can see that a

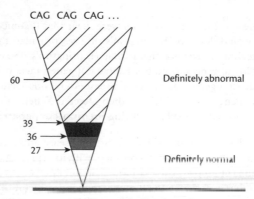

CAG CAG CAG ...

60 ——→ Definitely abnormal

39 ——→
36 ——→
27 ——→ Definitely normal

First part of the Huntington's gene

Figure 6.5 In 1998 the American College of Medical Genetics and the American Society of Human Genetics suggested ways in which the results of a genetic test should be reported. Under 27 repeats is clearly normal. Between 27 and 35 repeats (light grey band) the result is normal, but the repeat size may increase in future generations. Between 36 and 39 repeats inclusive (dark grey band), the result is abnormal. The individual might develop the condition very late or even not at all, but the children are still at risk. A result of 40 repeats and above is considered definitely abnormal.

few some individuals with results over 60 repeats started the disease later than 20 years and about half juvenile cases had results under 60 repeats. None the less, this is a useful rule of thumb.

Can you expect to be told your own repeat size?

There has been concern about the way the information about age of onset and repeat size can be interpreted for any particular individual. Some laboratories will report the actual repeat size, whereas others will only report the broad category result: normal, normal but in the 27 to 35 range, abnormal in the 36 to 39 range, or unequivocally abnormal. This gives the relevant clinical information and avoids misunderstandings on the part of either the doctor or the family. The laboratory with which I work reports the actual size in addition to the broad category. My own practice is not to discuss the actual repeat size with the patient or family unless I am specifically asked. If I am asked for the actual repeat size then I will check why the person has asked the question. I will tell them their repeat size, but also explain why the information is of limited value for an individual.

7

Genetic counselling: a new diagnosis in the family

> ➡ **Key points**
>
> ◆ Genetic counselling is a process of giving you information.
>
> ◆ Following a new diagnosis, issues that may be discussed include how the condition has affected you and your immediate family.
>
> ◆ It may take time to come to terms with a new diagnosis, but one aspect that needs to be tackled is letting close relatives know that they are now at increased risk of developing the condition.

If you, or a member of your family, has Huntington's disease then you will be offered genetic counselling. The offer may come from a hospital specialist around the time of diagnosis. Alternatively, you may initiate the referral yourself by asking your local doctor to refer you to the genetic clinic so that your questions can be answered. This could happen when a relative tells you that Huntington's disease is in the family; or it may be that, despite having known the family history for some time, you judge that it is now appropriate to get further information. Depending on your circumstances, you may go along to the genetic clinic as an individual, or else attend with your spouse or partner and have discussions as a couple.

The purpose of this chapter is to describe what is involved in genetic counselling in general terms and specifically for a couple in which one member is affected. Issues for predictive testing and prenatal tests will be considered in the next chapter.

Who are genetic counsellors and where do they work?

Usually, medical doctors lead genetic counselling teams. They are specially trained to give information about genetic disorders and explain the implications of genetic tests. The genetic tests are performed by scientific staff in the laboratory. It is unlikely that you will meet the scientists involved in analysing genetic tests of your family, but there are other members of the team with whom you may have a great deal of contact. These are non-medical genetic counsellors, who often have a background in nursing or related disciplines and are able to provide additional help and support.

Genetic conditions are rare, so genetic teams are usually located at large hospitals and serve a population of 2 to 4 million people. This does not necessarily mean that you have to travel to a large hospital, because the genetic teams hold clinics at local hospitals at regular intervals.

What is genetic counselling?

The main purpose of genetic counselling is to provide information about Huntington's disease (or, for that matter, other genetic disorders) so that individuals or couples can make informed choices. Genetic counselling should be considered as a process, which suggests that the information-giving may take place over a period of time. It is reasonable to ask how genetic counselling differs from any other medical consultation. Many medical consultations involve the doctor giving advice or recommending a particular form of treatment, whereas genetic counselling involves discussing options with you and then allowing you to decide the best way forward. It is not good enough to simply give information to people and say, 'Well, these are your options; now you choose'. The doctor or counsellor has to understand your particular circumstances and support you in a way that allows you to make your own decisions. Geneticists describe the process as 'non-directive' and 'non-judgmental'; this emphasizes the point that you are not told what to do. These general principles underlie all genetic counselling sessions, although each genetic counsellor has an individual style.

An essential step in any genetic counselling process is drawing a diagram of your family tree, such as the one shown in Figure 7.1. One reason for drawing the family tree is to provide an easy record of your family history. It also helps

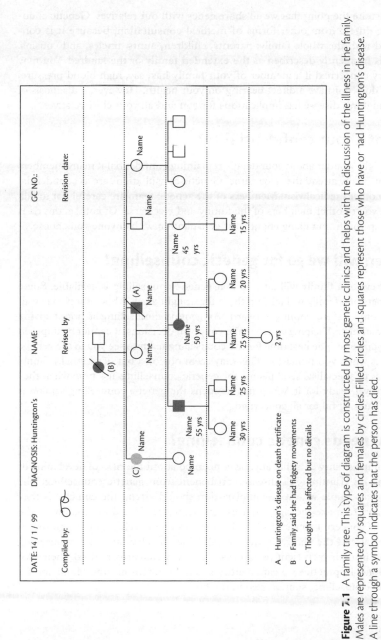

Figure 7.1 A family tree. This type of diagram is constructed by most genetic clinics and helps with the discussion of the illness in the family. Males are represented by squares and females by circles. Filled circles and squares represent those who have or had Huntington's disease. A line through a symbol indicates that the person has died.

DATE: 14 / 1 / 99   DIAGNOSIS: Huntington's   NAME: GC NO:

Compiled by: Revised by   Revision date:

A   Huntington's disease on death certificate

B   Family said she had fidgety movements

C   Thought to be affected but no details

71

to illustrate the point that we all share genes with our relatives. Genetic counselling differs from other forms of medical consultation, because it is concerned with the whole family: parents, children, aunts, uncles, and cousins. This is frequently described as the extended family or the kindred. You may be very concerned if a member of your family has, say, high blood pressure, but it does not have a direct bearing on your health. However, a diagnosis of Huntington's disease has implications for you and all your close relatives.

What about confidentiality?

You might wonder about your details remaining confidential if many members of your family attend the same clinic. Genetic consultations are as confidential as any other medical visit. Members of the genetic team are careful not to talk about you to other members of the family and vice versa. Of course, this does not stop you from talking about your consultation with anyone you choose.

When will we go for genetic counselling?

Members of a family will be told that genetic counselling is available. Some members of a family will take up the offer straight away, while others may wait some time before coming forward. As genetic counselling is about giving information and helping you to make your own decisions, it cannot be imposed by anyone else. The best time for the counselling team to see you in the genetic clinic is when you request it. This may seem obvious, but occasionally family doctors or specialists send people for genetic counselling at a time when they are not yet ready for it. When this happens the genetic counselling session is usually unhelpful for all concerned.

Who needs genetic counselling?

The simplest answer is that anyone concerned about the risks of developing or passing on Huntington's disease can benefit from genetic counselling. The person or couple who wants information should attend the clinic; it is they who have to make the right choices for themselves. You do not know all the issues of concern to an adult child, brother, sister, or even your partner, so you cannot attend the clinic on their behalf. They need to attend a counselling session in their own right to express their own concerns and ask their own questions. In practice we can identify several different groups who come for genetic counselling, summarized in the box.

> ❗ **Fact**
>
> There are different types of genetic counselling session:
>
> ◆ Those in which an individual or one member of a couple has already developed the condition;
>
> ◆ Those in which an individual or one member of a couple is at 50 per cent risk;
>
> ◆ Those in which an individual or one member of a couple is at 25 per cent risk.

The conversation you have with a genetic counsellor will vary depending on how new the diagnosis of Huntington's disease is to the family. The next section and the next chapter describes some of the issues that are discussed with each of these groups.

Genetic counselling for someone diagnosed with Huntington's disease

Several circumstances may result in genetic counselling being offered to someone with Huntington's disease (and their partner). An obvious time is when a diagnosis has just been made, and the family history has been either unknown or previously misunderstood. In this case you may experience a variety of emotions, but feelings of anger, anxiety, and frustration are all understandable. The counsellor may have to spend time with you going over information that was provided around the time of the diagnosis. This is because the shock you felt when you were given the diagnosis may have prevented you from understanding fully what was being said.

People frequently ask, 'Where has the disease come from?' As we saw in Chapter 6, a new diagnosis could be the result of a new mutation, but this is unusual. It is more likely that the family history has been unknown because of the early death of a parent, adoption, separation of the family, or the symptoms of Huntington's disease in an elderly parent going unrecognized. This last possibility could happen if one of your parents had been diagnosed with a neurological condition that has some of the features of Huntington's disease, such as Parkinson's disease or multiple sclerosis. This raises the suspicion that the correct diagnosis should have been Huntington's disease. Even if the diagnosis in one of your parents was Huntington's disease, it is possible that the genetic significance was either not properly explained, or, if it was, the family actively concealed the information so that it still comes as a shock to you. During the course of establishing the family history it may become obvious that other relatives are also similarly affected. They and their immediate family may then seek genetic counselling as a consequence.

It is almost inevitable that either you, or your partner, will ask about prospects for the future and methods of treatment. (The details of research and available treatments are explained in Chapters 2, 3, 10, and 11.) To some extent the answer will depend on your age and the stage of the illness at the time of diagnosis. Whilst it is important that questions are answered honestly, no-one can predict the future accurately. Replies often have to be of a general nature; phrases such as 'slowly progressive' are employed. Another way of talking about the course of the condition is to suggest that there is unlikely to be much difference in your condition from year to year, but people who know you may well notice a difference over a period of a few years.

If your family history is well known at the time of diagnosis, then discussions may turn on the way the condition was managed in the previous generation and the impact it had on you and your family. You may want to discuss practical issues such as driving and the ability to continue working; these have been discussed in Chapter 2.

Most people will have completed their family by the time a diagnosis of Huntington's disease is made, and their children will now be at risk of developing the disorder. Genetic counsellors will not make you tell your adult children about the condition. However, assuming that your children are adults, the diagnosis of Huntington's disease has implications for their health, the future health of their children (i.e. your grandchildren), and decisions they may be making about having or extending their own family. If you ask the question, 'Should we tell the children about Huntington's disease?' then a genetic counsellor may not answer directly but instead reply along the lines of, 'What are your concerns about talking to the children about Huntington's disease?'

Most parents worry about whether, and how, to tell children about a genetic problem. It may be very reasonable to take a little time to come to terms with a new diagnosis, but telling your children gives them options, including doing nothing, seeking information in their own right, deciding for themselves whether to extend their family, having a predictive test, or considering a prenatal test. These options are explained in more detail in the next chapter. Although it is understandable to feel that by not informing the children you are protecting them (particularly as there is no treatment to prevent or delay the onset of Huntington's disease), this is frequently not really the case. It is unlikely that you can conceal the diagnosis and genetic implications in the long term, as there is much more publicity about Huntington's disease in the media and in schools than there has been in the past. If your children do find out about Huntington's disease some other way they will probably feel angry on the grounds that they should have been given the opportunity to make their own informed choices. Whilst finding out about Huntington's disease can never be good news, it is my experience that people do not like being kept in the dark about issues that directly affect them.

If your children are young, then time is available to consider the best method of informing them. There is no 'right' way of explaining the issues to children. Parents sometimes feel they must wait until the 'right' time. Putting off a discussion until school examinations are over, or until the child has grown up and is in a steady relationship, has the disadvantage that the information may come as a shock. Another disadvantage is that the child may well guess some of the implications, but, sensing a family secret, feels unable to discuss them with you. Whilst it is not possible to be dogmatic about the 'right' age to tell children, many parents feel that it is best to start feeding them some information at an early age. It is possible to encourage children to ask questions and then to give answers that are appropriate for their age and understanding. Over time the children grow up knowing that one parent has Huntington's disease and knowing the implications for themselves. It comes as less of a shock, family relationships are easier to maintain, and, in due course, the children are able to make their own decisions about how to deal with their risk.

An essential component of the genetic counselling process is to offer support. You need to feel that you can contact the clinic again, as and when necessary. In this context, you need to know that further help and information is available when either you or your children request it. The counsellor may give you the address of a patients' organization. No-one is forced to join, but you have the option of making contact if and when you are ready. Patients' organizations have leaflets and booklets which, among other things, can help you come to terms with knowing your own diagnosis, caring for a relative with Huntington's disease, or telling your children about the condition.

Similar considerations apply to telling your brothers and sisters and other relatives about the diagnosis. Occasionally, difficulties with relationships in a family mean that giving information takes time. It is better for genetic counsellors to work with families rather than force issues and impose genetic counselling on them, as this is likely to be counter-productive. Genetic counsellors are frequently able to maintain contact with some members of either your close or extended family, so in most cases, and over time, they can be sure that relevant members of your extended family are aware of the diagnosis of Huntington's disease. In this way your other relatives are able to choose whether and when to seek further help and information

Research

You may ask about prospects for research to improve treatment. This is considered in more detail in Chapter 11. Not everyone wants to participate in research projects, but others will consider this for a number of reasons: perhaps, in part, because it is an opportunity to do something positive, or perhaps from a desire to see an improvement for children and grandchildren. The development of research networks as described in Chapter 11 makes it easier to access involvement in research projects.

Conclusion

Genetic counselling is a process that involves information-giving and support. The issues discussed will vary depending on whether or not you or a spouse or partner has the condition, and on whether you are unaffected but at risk. This chapter has focused on issues for coming to terms with a new diagnosis and letting other family members know that they are now at increased risk.

8

Genetic counselling for unaffected family members

> ⊃ **Key points**

- Options for individuals at risk for Huntington's disease include not having a genetic test, having a predictive test, and having a test in pregnancy.

- There are no treatments to delay the onset of Huntington's disease or to slow down the damage to nerve cells in the brain once the condition has started.

- Approximately 20 per cent of individuals at risk for Huntington's disease choose to have a test to see whether they will or will not develop the condition at some time in the future.

There may be many reasons for choosing a test, but the ones given to me most frequently are that certainty is better than uncertainty, and the need to give information to children. This is a common reason for referral. You may have known about the risks of Huntington's disease in the family for some time and now feel you want more information about the genetic aspects of Huntington's disease for a variety of reasons. You might have heard about genetic tests, have plans for marriage or starting a family, or want to talk to your children and need to know about yourself first. Alternatively, you may have discovered the risks of Huntington's disease following a new diagnosis in your parent. In either case, you may attend the clinic alone or, as is more usual, attend as a couple in which one partner has an affected parent. The nature of the discussion will vary depending on the particular circumstances. However, specific aspects of the counselling are given below.

Risk estimation

As Huntington's disease is inherited in an autosomal dominant manner (see Chapter 5 for further details), anyone with an affected parent has a 50 per cent chance of inheriting the disease. As we saw in Chapter 1, the disease often starts between the ages of 35 years and 55 years, so as you become older and remain well it is less likely that you have inherited the gene. If you have an affected parent and are well at a particular age, then it is possible to work out the chance that you will develop Huntington's disease in the future. At the age of 20 years this is still very close to 50 per cent; this is called your prior risk, but as you go through your mid-forties this chance is approximately 33 per cent; this is called your residual or age modified risk. An important point is that, even if you are well at 70 years old and over, there is still a small chance that you could have the gene. The identification of the Huntington's disease gene in 1993 made predictive testing much easier. Before 1993 a lot of time was spent explaining this residual risk to family members. This may still be important for some people but more often discussion focuses on the use of the predictive test. Given this shift in emphasis, I will not give the detail of how this residual risk, or age modified risk, is estimated from the age at onset curve.

People with a prior risk of 50 per cent sometimes ask if their children can develop Huntington's disease before them. Although some very exceptional cases have been described in the medical literature where this may have happened, it is possible to be reassuring on this point: in the overwhelming majority of cases children do not develop features of Huntington's disease ahead of a parent at 50 per cent risk.

Telling the children about Huntington's disease

Many people who discover that they have a 50 per cent prior risk (i.e. have an affected parent) will have young children. If this is the case, you and your partner have to decide when and how to tell the children about Huntington's disease being in the family. The general issues and principles involved have been discussed in the previous chapter. Some people decide to talk openly about Huntington's disease within the family so that their children are used to the family history of Huntington's disease from an early age. Many people have told me about their experiences of discussing the implications of

Huntington's disease with their children and I have been struck by the acceptance and resilience of young people.

Options available

Before describing the predictive test in great detail it may be helpful to comment that although there are a variety of options available, there is no perfect solution: each option has a drawback. The important point is that you choose the option that is right for you

Not having a predictive test

For many people, accepting the risk is the most appropriate option. This has the drawback that you may still worry about the risk. If you have children and develop the condition later in life they will be at 50 per cent risk. For the reasons given above, as you get older and stay well the chance of you developing Huntington's disease in the future starts to reduce, but this reduction is not dramatic until after the usual years of reproduction. Many individuals and couples decide not to have children for all sorts of different reasons. Not having children might be acceptable but has the drawback that you could discover much later in life that you are unaffected. If you do not want a predictive test then it is still possible to have children who will be free of risk. Obviously for a male partner who is at risk, this could involve using donor sperm. This has the obvious drawback that you are not the biological father of the child. In my experience, this option is not pursued very often.

Exclusion testing in pregnancy

If you have decided that a predictive test is not an option for you then it is still possible to have an **exclusion test in pregnancy**. This allows you to have your own children but to test a pregnancy in such a way that the risk of Huntington's disease is excluded, without altering your own risk. The obvious disadvantage to this is that it might involve one or more terminations of pregnancy. A variation of this method is to apply the same technique to preimplantation genetic diagnosis (PGD). Although this might seem a worthwhile alternative, it involves complicated *in vitro* fertilization (IVF) techniques, which has the disadvantage of being a complex procedure with a success rate of one chance in three. I will discuss the options of exclusion testing and the PGD variation in the section on pregnancy testing.

ⓘ Patient's perspective

I am grateful for this personal story about being at risk for Huntington's disease. Not unreasonably, the author does not want to be identified. Each person makes their own decision about how they cope with being at risk, but it may be helpful to record this example of a real experience.

"In many ways I am a typical 27-year-old, though it is sometimes hard to remember that. I have always been independent (my family might argue I am just stubborn) and I do take pride in doing my own thing and not following the crowd. One question I will never be able to answer is what different life choices I would have made if I had not been hit by the bombshell of the news we had HD in our family when I was 17. At that stage I had only come across HD as a hypothetical disease whilst learning about the statistics of genetics during my biology A-level. We were fortunate to have a fantastic GP who took the time to talk to us and answer as many of our questions as he could after hours in the local surgery. Looking back I can't remember how long it took for the idea to become reality for me, and to be honest there are probably still times when it feels like it's all happening to someone else, like I am watching some cheesy TV movie which seems just too tragic to be real.

The other lucky break was having the strength and support of my family; there were three of us in the surgery that evening, all reacting in our different ways (I clearly remember being the only one that burst into tears—younger sister's prerogative maybe) and now, though we are much further apart, I still draw huge support from knowing that they are both there whenever I need to talk, or just have a hug (it's always worth the train fare for that). We have been through so much together and it is a great relief to have people who know the whole story already—I don't need to explain from the beginning.

Which brings me to my most recent musings on 'the whole HD thing', which for the vast majority of the time is just another thing that might happen one day, like being hit by a bus or getting cancer—all those things that only happen to other people. What brings it all to life and makes it feel real is talking to people about it. At the moment I am not using any of the HD Association's support group network, but I am glad to know it is there. This last year has been a time of change and happiness, as I was completely surprised to meet someone in the summer who has become very important to me, and of course it is impossible to dream about future happiness with the HD cloud following me around. The questions soon arise: how soon do I have to risk shattering our happiness by telling you about this? How much can I expect you to understand in one go? Is it even reasonable to load my problem onto your shoulders (though I can't say I wouldn't appreciate having someone to share the weight some days)? One of the main difficulties is balancing the emotional issues surrounding my potential future and the practicalities of my fears above and beyond the 'normal' avoidance of unwanted pregnancies. It is impossible to talk about even a simple thing like contraception without going into the whole business of the science, the medicine, and the family history—all adding up to a not very romantic scenario!

So it was all a bit terrifying, but I have lived to tell the tale; it was never going to be easy but I could only live a few weeks with it all pressing on my mind and so jumped in with both feet with an awful 'There is something I have to tell you . . .' or something equally clichéd. I don't remember my exact words but I do remember the relief and the joy of being hugged and understood and that he didn't run away. We haven't been through it all yet and I know there are still questions but it gives me great hope that we are strong enough together to talk about them. If we can get through this obstacle then why should anything worry us? Maybe there are some positives to the whole HD thing. It has made me feel more secure; now for a while at least I can just concentrate on being happy."

Storing DNA

After discussion, you may come to the conclusion that you do not want a predictive test but would rather leave a sample of DNA in storage at the testing centre so that it is available for analysis after your death for the benefit of your children. It would also be available for analysis in the future if you change your mind about a predictive test. When your children are adults they can have a test in their own right, but if you die early it would be easier to test your sample because if it is negative your children do not need any further tests. If it is positive then each child can decide whether or not to have tests for themselves. I have included this option for completeness, although I have not had a request for this for some years.

Predictive testing

Predictive testing is a method of determining whether an individual has inherited the Huntington's disease gene *before* the onset of the disease.

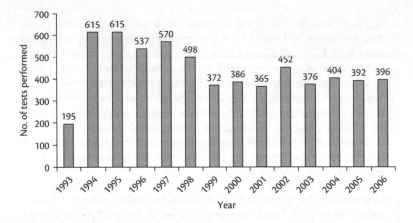

Figure 8.1 Bar chart showing the number of predictive tests for Huntington's disease undertaken in British genetic centres, 1993–2005. See text for an explanation. Figure courtesy of the UK Huntington's Disease Predictive Test Consortium.

Several different types of predictive test were considered in the past but there were doubts about their reliability and so they were never used. The current test examines the genetic material directly and is therefore much more reliable. A number of centres from Britain have kept records of the number of tests performed each year since the gene was identified in 1993 (Fig. 8.1). There is a trend, with not many tests being done in the first year because the technique was brand-new. More tests were undertaken in the early years that the test was available, suggesting there were a number of people wanting, and waiting for, such a test to become available. More recently, the trend has been for just under 400 tests to be done each year. Whilst it is possible to count the number of people having a predictive test each year, it is less easy to know how many people choose not to be tested. Estimates suggest that approximately 80 per cent of people at risk choose not to be tested.

Guidelines for predictive testing

There are international guidelines for predictive testing, so before describing what is involved in a predictive test, we need to consider why these guidelines were established.

Need for guidelines

When predictive testing first became a real possibility, there was concern that people might have their blood tested without first having genetic counselling. There was also a worry about the potential misuse of the information by others in society. The basic problem is that if someone has a positive result, it indicates that he or she will develop a progressive neurological illness at some time in the future, for which no effective treatment is available. Therefore, there is no direct advantage in medical terms in knowing that you carry the gene. In addition, there were fears that people would take the test without thinking through the implications and regret the decision afterwards.

An international committee composed of members of the World Federation of Neurology Research Group on Huntington's disease and members from the International Huntington's Association, which is the patients' organization, prepared the guidelines. Although the members of this group were selected, it is interesting to note that they were drawn from among scientists and doctors active in research and representatives of patient groups. These guidelines do not have the force of law but establish a framework for doctors from different countries to provide predictive tests in a consistent way. Guidelines cannot cover every situation, but they do help to set out the basic principles. In addition, they form the basis for further discussion, and unlike laws can be modified easily in the light of experience or new information. The description of the predictive test that follows is based on those guidelines.

Counselling aspects

The guidelines clearly state that anyone having a predictive test needs a minimum of two counselling sessions, separated by at least one month. In practice there may be more than a month between the two sessions. At first glance this seems dictatorial; therefore, it is important for you to understand some of the areas that will be discussed. It is my experience that the majority of people coming forward for a predictive test have already reached the decision that they would prefer to know whether or not they have the gene rather than remain 'at risk'. This means that the discussion is often not about whether or not you want to be tested but about making sure that the consequences have been considered fully.

Topics that may be covered before having a predictive test

You (and your partner) and the counsellor need the chance to think through the implications of a positive test result as well as a negative result. Each counsellor is different, but you will probably be asked why you think the test is in your best interest. There may be a mixture of reasons why you are considering a predictive test but people often say that they need to know for themselves; that is, certainty is better than uncertainty. This is certainly the most common reason given to me. You may also want definite information so that you know what to say to your children or to help you decide about starting a family. You may be asked how you and your family will feel if the test shows you have the gene and how you will feel if the test shows you do not have the gene. In fact, neither you nor anyone else can say exactly how you will react to being told that you will develop Huntington's disease in the future, or conversely that you are no longer at risk. The counsellor can tell you how other couples have reacted and can tell you the results of studies of predictive testing in the medical literature. However, the counsellor cannot say how *you* will react. In general, the number of adverse effects, in terms of serious depression or suicide, has been few. It is possible that these severe reactions were due to the onset of the disease coinciding with the test result.

It is natural for anyone receiving bad news to feel upset or down for a time, but most individuals or couples recover over a relatively short period. One reason to have your partner present during the predictive testing sessions is to provide support for you; however, it may be the case that your partner is more upset if the result indicates that you are going to develop Huntington's disease, as your partner also has to come to terms with a sense of loss. Some people at risk of Huntington's disease have come to terms with the idea of developing the condition in the future, so in a sense the result of the predictive test is not new to them; this is often not the case for their partner.

You might expect that if the result indicates that you have not inherited the gene then that is good news. Indeed it is, but some people have felt guilty that they have escaped, whereas other members of their family have not. Some people have been a little frustrated because they spent years worrying needlessly about Huntington's disease. After the relief of knowing that you have not got the gene you will have to come back to the reality of dealing with common worries such as jobs, money, and relationships, but at least you will know that you and your children will not get Huntington's disease.

Other areas for discussion could include possible effects on any children, as a positive result will mean that their prior risks are automatically elevated from 25 per cent to 50 per cent. Depending on the circumstances, it may be appropriate to discuss the possibility of prenatal tests. Similarly it may be relevant for an individual or couple to consider the effect of a positive predictive test result on any future insurance proposal or other legal contract.

Special circumstances may arise if the counsellor is worried that someone is already showing signs of depression. If this happens then there may be a need to consider postponing the test until a psychiatrist or general practitioner has had an opportunity to ensure that treatment for depression and additional support are available. Another area of difficulty is when the counsellor detects the early clinical signs of the disease but the person seeking the test is seemingly unaware of them. If the counsellor is confident about the clinical signs then it is inevitable that the test will be positive. One way of dealing with this is to ask if the individual or their partner is worried that Huntington's disease has already started. Another way is to ask if the person would like to be examined and know the results of a clinical neurological examination, after which any suspicions can be discussed.

Your counsellor will spend time describing the technical aspects of the test. Some centres ask for a written consent form to be signed before blood is taken for the test. The signed consent form confirms in writing the major points that were discussed. The counsellor will also need to discuss the manner in which the result will be delivered. The guidelines are specific: this should be done in person and not via the telephone or by letter. The counsellor will also explain the arrangements for professional support when you receive the result. The guidelines are clear that testing centres should have the ability to provide counselling and support after the test result. You will also want to think about which relatives and friends you will tell as part of your own general mechanism of support. Some people have chosen to discuss the results with their employers, whereas others would never consider this. Testing centres are very concerned that confidentiality should be the rule. The results of a predictive test should not be disclosed to anyone else without your permission but it is customary for your family doctor to be informed. This has the obvious advantage that your family doctor can be part of the support mechanism. Very occasionally, I have had requests that the family doctor should not be informed. Rather than refuse, I have taken time to explore why the person does not want this to happen.

Given the need to have a wide-ranging discussion and to impart technical information, it is not surprising that more than one session is required. Although some people complain that this prolongs the testing procedure, it has the advantage that you have been able to discuss all the issues, some of which you may not have considered previously. You have the opportunity to think about both the advantages and disadvantages of the test so your final decision is informed. Taking two sessions also means that your decision has been consistent over a period of time; this is especially important for those who have only recently learnt that they are at risk because of a new diagnosis in the family, as a decision to go ahead with the test when you may be shocked or angry needs to be considered carefully. If more sessions are needed then these will be arranged.

The majority of people will have their predictive test according to the guidelines but they can be modified in exceptional circumstances. An obvious exception might be someone coming to the clinic when they are already several weeks pregnant. Providing genetic counselling when a pregnancy is underway is always less than ideal because decisions about tests have to be taken quickly if they are to influence whether or not to continue the pregnancy.

Finally, the age at which someone can have a predictive test needs to be considered. The guidelines state that the person should have reached the age of majority for the relevant country. In the UK this is 18 years, which can cause confusion because individuals can normally give consent for medical procedures after the age of 16 years. The intention behind the guideline is that the person should be mature. Judging maturity is very difficult: a teenager could be very mature, whereas someone aged 20 or 21 could be less mature. In any event there is no intention to test children. This rule does protect children but can cause difficulties if a child or young teenager has behavioural problems (see Chapter 4).

Technical aspects of the test

As part of the process of ensuring informed choice, you need to understand some of the technical aspects of the laboratory test. It may be easiest to begin with basics and remind you that we have two copies of our genes and that they are packaged onto chromosomes (see Chapter 5 for further details). The gene for Huntington's disease is on chromosome 4. Your affected parent has one normal copy of the gene and one that causes Huntington's disease. The copy of the gene that causes Huntington's disease has a part which is larger than normal. You are bound to have a normal-sized copy of the gene from your unaffected parent. The question is: did you inherit the normal-sized copy from your affected parent, in which case Huntington's disease will not develop or did you inherit the larger copy, in which case you will develop Huntington's disease at some time in the future? The chance that the result will be positive, that is, that the Huntington's disease has been inherited, is based on your age-modified risk, already described. If you are in your twenties this is still effectively 50 per cent, but if you are aged 45 years it is 33 per cent and if you are older it will be even lower (see page 78).

If you decide to go ahead then your genetic material will be extracted from a sample of blood. It is a relatively easy laboratory procedure to assess the sizes of the genes (see Chapter 6). In the majority of cases the results are clearcut, with either two normal-sized copies of the gene present (a good news or negative result) or one normal and one large result (a bad news or positive result).

Although no medical test can be described as 100 per cent accurate, the chances of error involved in direct tests of the gene are extremely small, but difficult to calculate. The test can be described as close to 100 per cent accurate. It is my practice to ask the laboratory to process two samples of blood separately in the hope that this will prevent people worrying 'Did they get it right?' at a later date. As a further precaution, the testing centre may check that a positive test result has been obtained on an affected member of your family. Checking that an affected relative has a positive result does remove the, admittedly remote, possibility that Huntington's disease is not the correct diagnosis.

As we saw on page 60, the size of the gene is unhelpful in predicting the age of onset for any particular person. In order to prevent confusion some centres will not tell you the exact size of the gene but just give the result as positive or negative.

Results in the grey area

In fact, there are two grey areas to consider. The first is a result in the range of 36 to 39 repeats and the second is a result in the range of 27 to 35 repeats (see Fig. 6.5).

On page 65, I explained that in exceptional cases someone with a repeat size in the range of 36 to 39 repeats could develop Huntington's disease at the usual time, or very late in life, or even have died as an elderly person before the condition started. If the result of a predictive test is in this range then a genetic counsellor may have to explain this possibility to you, but also emphasize that your children would still be at risk of developing Huntington's disease. If you have a predictive test result in this range, then one way of explaining that you may not develop the condition is to say there is at least a 40 per cent chance you will develop the condition after the age of 65 years and at least a 30 per cent chance you will develop it after 75 years.

A different grey area is the result in the range of 27 to 35 repeats. If you have this result then it is clear that you yourself will not develop Huntington's disease, but there are still potential implications for your descendants. The problem is that when Huntington's disease starts for the first time as a new mutation in the family, the unaffected parent has had a result in this range. There must be a lot of people in the population who have a result in this range and it is passed from generation to generation without a problem. The issue is that, although the chance of Huntington's disease affecting your descendants is very small, it cannot be totally excluded. This result is often disappointing because you cannot completely reassure your children that the family history of Huntington's disease is no longer relevant. Depending on what your children think, they can come forward for testing to make sure that the gene size has not increased in them. This has the advantage that they get information in their own right.

Given that grey area results occur infrequently, I often warn people coming for testing that occasionally we may get a result that is difficult to interpret, but do not go into great detail unless it occurs.

Predictive tests and insurance

A fundamental principle of an insurance policy is that you and the company act in good faith. This means that you have to declare all relevant information about yourself at the time you take out insurance. If you took out a policy and answered the questions honestly before finding out about Huntington's disease, then you need have no concern. If the family history of Huntington's disease is known, then the insurance company can take this into account when setting the premium. There has been a concern that healthy individuals with positive predictive test results would have great difficulty obtaining new insurance policies. In the UK, the government and insurance companies have agreed a moratorium. In essence, this means that the result of a positive predictive test will be ignored for most forms of insurance, but the premium will still be based on the family history. Insurance companies do accept the result of a negative test and offer premiums at standard rates based on your age, whether you smoke, and any other health problems you may have. This moratorium will last until 2011 but is due for reconsideration shortly. During counselling for a predictive test I mention the issue of insurance and suggest that if an individual or couple would like more advice then the testing process can be deferred until they have had an opportunity to obtain independent financial advice. In my experience, most people have already decided that a predictive test is the way forward and insurance is not a major issue. Other countries have different social structures and have taken other approaches to this problem.

Prenatal testing

Prenatal diagnosis is a method of detecting in the early stages of pregnancy whether a fetus has, or has not, inherited the Huntington's disease gene.

As with predictive testing, the issues involved have to be considered carefully. If you know you have inherited the gene as a result of a predictive test (or possibly because of the onset of the condition), you might want to think about prenatal diagnosis. If cells of fetal origin are obtained early in the course of a pregnancy then the same laboratory techniques described previously may be used to determine whether the fetus has inherited the Huntington's disease gene. If the result is negative then the decision to continue the pregnancy is straightforward. Alternatively, if the result is positive then you have to consider termination of the pregnancy. Termination of a wanted pregnancy is obviously very traumatic and needs to be discussed sensitively. An important point to realize is that if the result is positive and you then refuse a termination, the child will be born with the certainty of developing Huntington's disease in the future. If this happens, then the child will grow up with the knowledge that he or she is going to develop Huntington's disease and will have been denied the opportunity to decide for him or herself whether to have the test as an adult. Ideally, the counsellor will discuss these issues well before a pregnancy so that you are able to come to terms with the possible outcomes of a prenatal test.

Apart from the genetic aspects of prenatal diagnosis, the obstetric aspects must also be considered; these are essentially the same whatever the genetic condition. There are two common methods of obtaining fetal cells: the first is called **chorion biopsy** (another name is chorionic villus biopsy or CVS) and the second is called **amniocentesis**. Each of these obstetric procedures has advantages and disadvantages. Chorion biopsy involves taking a small piece of the placenta or afterbirth at about 10 to 11 weeks into the pregnancy, as shown in Figure 8.2. There are two ways of reaching the placenta, depending on its position within the uterus. One is to pass a catheter through the vagina and neck of the womb; the other method involves passing a needle through the skin of the abdomen. Most chorion biopsies are done by passing a needle through the skin. Whichever method is chosen, an ultrasound scan guides the obstetrician to the correct place. It is very important to realize that the needle or catheter is not put into the fetus. The biopsy will contain both fetal and maternal tissue; the maternal tissue can be stripped away in the laboratory, leaving enough fetal tissue for the DNA test. The result should be available before the twelfth week of the pregnancy. If you require a termination, this can be undertaken by inducing a miscarriage with tablets and a pessary or using a general anaesthetic. If this need arises you can discuss the different methods with the obstetric team.

One disadvantage of the procedure is that it could cause a miscarriage to occur in a pregnancy that would otherwise continue. Each antenatal clinic

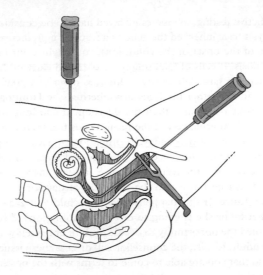

Figure 8.2 The technique of chorion biopsy. In this procedure the obstetrician wants to obtain cells from the placenta or afterbirth. There are two ways of approaching the placenta. One way is through the neck of the womb and the other is through the skin of the abdomen. Both approaches are shown in the diagram but of course only one would be chosen. Nowadays the approach through the skin is chosen most often. In either case an ultrasound machine is used to help guide the obstetrician.

quotes slightly different risk figures but approximately 2 per cent (2 in 100) is reasonable. This can be broken down into about a 1 per cent background chance of miscarriage and an extra 1 per cent chance due to the procedure. The procedure can also be done later in the pregnancy, but most couples find it possible to contact an appropriate centre soon after a pregnancy has been confirmed. The advantages of obtaining results in the first three months of pregnancy include having a test when knowledge of the pregnancy can still be private to the couple concerned, and that if there is a need to have a termination it can be performed either surgically or inducing a miscarriage medically with tablets and a pessary.

The alternative procedure, amniocentesis, involves taking some fluid from around the 'baby' at approximately 16 weeks. This fluid contains some fetal cells, which can be grown in culture and used in the DNA test. Although the risk of miscarriage is said to be about 1 per cent (compared to 2 per cent for chorion biopsy) the test result is available later in the pregnancy; if you require a termination this would only be done by inducing a miscarriage medically. The majority of couples opt for the earlier test.

Exclusion testing in pregnancy

The description of the discovery of the Huntington's disease gene is given in Chapter 5. An essential step was the discovery, in 1983, that the gene for Huntington's disease is on chromosome 4, although its precise position was not known until 1993. There were a series of markers, or variations in the DNA, close to the gene, which could be traced through a family in order to provide genetic information to those at risk. Essentially, these markers are present in every family and by themselves are not useful. However, in a family with Huntington's disease, if a specific marker was shown to be inherited with the gene then predictive information was obtained for those at risk. The main problem with this type of test was that it required a family study of at least two and ideally three generations. In practice, most Huntington's disease families were too small to make use of the technology. One application was, and remains, the exclusion test in pregnancy. In this analysis the three generations are made up from a couple with one partner at 50 per cent risk, the parent of the at-risk person, and the fetus, as shown in Figure 8.3. In the example, the person at risk inherited marker A from his affected parent and marker B from his unaffected parent. By itself this gives no extra information except to say

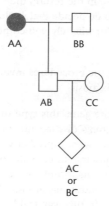

Figure 8.3 Diagram to illustrate an exclusion test in pregnancy. The markers **A**, **B**, and **C** represent natural variations in the DNA molecule close to the Huntington's disease gene. The way of working out whether the risk to the fetus has increased or decreased is given in the text.

that marker A is associated with the risk of Huntington's disease and marker B is not. If the fetus inherits marker B then it has inherited the chromosome 4 from its unaffected grandparent; therefore, Huntington's disease has been excluded. Conversely, if the fetus inherits marker A the risk has increased from 25 per cent to 50 per cent. Huntington's disease has not been excluded but equally it is not definite that the fetus will develop Huntington's disease. The parent's risk has not altered; the only question being asked in this test is, 'Did the fetus inherit the chromosome 4 that came from its affected grandparent or did it inherit the chromosome 4 from its unaffected grandparent?' As this is an indirect method of studying the gene there is a small error associated with the test, of the order of 1 per cent. Another point to realize is that if Huntington's disease is not excluded, the at-risk parent and the fetus have inherited the same chromosome 4 from the affected grandparent and now have the same genetic risks (barring the small error because the test is indirect).

If the fetus has inherited the chromosome 4 from its affected grandparent and is now at 50 per cent risk, you now have a difficult decision regarding termination of the pregnancy. Both you and the fetus share the same chromosome as the affected grandparent. If you continue the pregnancy and at some point in the future you develop Huntington's disease, it will be clear that your child is also going to be affected. Your child will then grow up knowing he or she is going to develop Huntington's disease rather than just being at risk. The child will have had no opportunity to decide for him or herself whether to be tested as an adult. On the other hand, if you terminate the pregnancy and do not develop Huntington's disease in the future, then you will know that the child would not have either. If you do decide that exclusion testing is a good option for you, the genetic counsellor will help you come to terms with these choices prior to a pregnancy.

The description of the obstetric procedures involved is the same as that given in the section on prenatal diagnosis.

Since the identification of the gene, this type of test is less relevant to most couples at risk for Huntington's disease; however, it is occasionally considered when someone does not want a predictive test but does want children free from risk, and artificial insemination by donor or pre-implantation genetic diagnosis are unacceptable or inappropriate. It has to be said that this test is complex and still provokes controversy among doctors, because, on average, half of all pregnancies tested in this way will be terminated on the basis of a 50 per cent risk, which means that half the fetuses terminated will not have inherited the gene.

Pre-implantation genetic diagnosis

The genetic test will work on any tissue that contains cells. In recent years pre-implantation genetic diagnosis (PGD) has become more widely discussed. The technique can be used either for direct testing and then implanting only those embryos that have the normal-sized copy of the gene, or for exclusion testing if the at-risk partner does not want to alter his or her own risk status. Although this sounds like a neat way of getting around the issue of termination of pregnancy, it is still a very complex procedure, which may be very demanding for the couple concerned. Essentially, the female partner takes drugs to suppress her ovaries. This is followed by drugs to stimulate the ovaries. Once this is done, an ultrasound scan can assess how many eggs can be harvested from the ovaries. Harvesting the eggs is done in an operating theatre. Once the eggs are obtained, they can be fertilized outside the womb with sperm from the male partner and the embryo grown to about the eight-cell stage. One or two cells can be taken and used to perform a genetic test (either a direct test or an exclusion test). Only those embryos that are not at risk are suitable for re-implantation. In general terms, the success rate of taking a baby home after this procedure is approximately one chance in five at the start of the process and about one chance in three once suitable embryos are available. As you might expect, the success rate falls if the female partner is in her late thirties or early forties. Another disadvantage is the cost. Pre-implantation genetic diagnosis is more expensive than ordinary IVF and, depending on the country in which you live, you may or may not be eligible for help with the cost. In the UK, not all couples are eligible for PGD from the National Health Service. This should be seen as a complex option, which may be pursued by a few couples.

Genetic counselling for an individual at 25 per cent risk

The identification of the gene means that genetic tests no longer require complex family studies. Anyone with an affected grandparent but with an unaffected parent (who has not had or does not want a predictive test) may request a test for themselves. If you are in this position it is now technically possible to have a test, but in addition to the general points about predictive testing the counsellor will want to discuss the effects of the result on the rest of the family. Clearly, if you are shown to have the gene then your unaffected parent must also have the gene and your brothers and sisters will be at 50 per cent risk. On the other hand, if you do not have the gene then other family members cannot infer any information about themselves. This is because it is still possible for the gene to be present in your at-risk parent. Unless there has been complete fragmentation of the family, it is unlikely that you could keep a positive result completely secret. The counsellor will ask whether it is possible for you to tell your at-risk parent what you are planning before the test is carried out. It is obviously up to you whether you have the test but your counsellor will want to know that you have thought through the impact of the test on your family.

Conclusion

Genetic counselling is a process that allows you to obtain accurate information about Huntington's disease. The counsellor wants to help you come to terms with the fact that Huntington's disease has occurred in your family and give you time to choose your best option, given your particular circumstances. Although much has been made of recent developments in predictive testing this option is only pursued by a minority of those at risk.

The localization of the Huntington's disease to chromosome 4 and its subsequent identification has increased the range of options available for people at risk for Huntington's disease. The initial fears that there would be major adverse effects of predictive testing precipitated a dialogue between professionals interested in Huntington's disease and the lay organizations, which resulted in the development of guidelines. Although individuals select themselves for predictive testing there have been few serious adverse effects, which may in part be due to the careful genetic counselling accompanying the test. It needs to be emphasized that identifying the gene for Huntington's disease was not an end in itself, nor was its purpose solely to develop predictive tests or tests in pregnancy. The objective was, and remains, to increase the basic understanding of Huntington's disease in the hope that this will lead to more effective treatment.

9

Changes in the brain

⊃ Key points

◆ Certain parts of the brain are affected more obviously than others.

◆ The most obvious damage to the brain occurs to groups of cells at the base of the brain called the caudate and putamen nuclei.

◆ Even in the caudate and putamen nuclei, some nerve cells are more susceptible to damage from the abnormal huntingtin than others. The explanation for this remains unclear.

◆ Less obvious damage occurs in some other parts of the brain.

As you might expect, the changes that occur in the brain of someone with Huntington's disease have been studied in great detail over many years. In this chapter I want to describe this pattern of change. It is interesting in itself, but will also help in understanding some ideas for further research, which will be described in the next chapter.

What is a nerve cell?

The brain contains millions of nerve cells, or **neurons**. Figure 9.1 shows a diagram of a typical nerve cell or neurons. It consists of a main area called the **nerve cell body**, which is covered in **projections** or **dendrites**. Most of the projections are small and these receive impulses from other nerve cells. There is one larger projection, called an **axon**, which may or may not be covered in fatty material. This axon transmits impulses to another part of the nervous system. A nerve cell receives an impulse because a chemical is transmitted from the end of one nerve cell to one of the projections on the other cell. If the

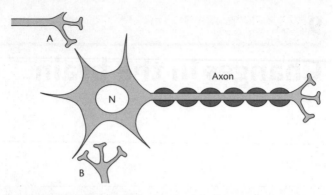

Figure 9.1 The parts of a nerve cell. The genetic material is found in the nucleus (**N**). The main part of the nerve cell is covered in projections or dendrites so that it can receive chemical messages from other nerve cells (represented as **A** and **B**). The nerve cell has a long projection called an axon, which may or may not be covered with fatty material. The nerve can transmit impulses to another part of the nervous system via chemical messages from the end of the axon.

nerve cell bodies are collected together in an area of the brain it will have a grey colour, whereas areas of the brain that contain the long projections covered in fatty material appear white.

Are there any changes to be seen on just looking at the brain?

One of the first things a doctor will notice when looking at the brain of someone who has died after many years of Huntington's disease is that the brain is slightly smaller and weighs a little less, and the folds on the surface are a little wider than the brain of someone the same age who died of something completely different, say a heart attack. This change could occur in a lot of neurological disorders, and further work needs to be done to recognize the pattern of changes typical of Huntington's disease.

Are there changes to be seen when the brain is cut?

If the brain is cut into, the pattern of damage becomes apparent. If you look at the picture of the normal brain in Figure 9.2 you can see that there is grey matter around the outside and white matter in the middle. The grey matter around the outside of the brain is called the **cortex**. At the base of the brain more grey matter can be seen. This area of grey matter contains more nerve

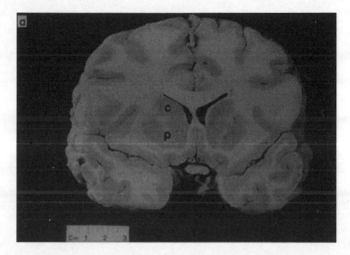

Figure 9.2 Photograph of a cut brain from an individual who did not have Huntington's disease. The surface of the brain is called the cortex and is grey because nerve cells are present here. The fatty material on the axons makes the brain appear white. There is another large area of grey in the middle of the picture (labelled C and P), which is the basal ganglia. This figure was published in Huntington's Dicsease, Ed Harper PS, 1991, page 145. Copyright Elsevier.

cells and is called the **basal ganglia** (labelled C and P). In this section of the brain it is in two parts, which are called the **caudate nucleus** and the **putamen**. The shape of the basal ganglia is important. The caudate nucleus bulges into what appears to be a space. (In life this space is filled with fluid.)

If you now look at a similar section of the brain of someone who died of Huntington's disease (Fig. 9.3), you can see that the folds on the surface are wider, but more importantly the basal ganglia are reduced to a rim of tissue. You can see that after many years of Huntington's disease there is considerable damage to the basal ganglia. In fact, similar changes can be seen on a brain scan during life, as shown in Figure 9.4.

As we saw in Chapter 6, we now have a very reliable genetic test. Before the genetic test was available, pathologists were asked to examine the brains of people who had died of an illness that could have been Huntington's disease. The question arose as to whether the pathologist could give an absolutely definite diagnosis. The answer to this was 'not quite'. Pathologists act in much the same way as other doctors when making a diagnosis: they try to recognize particular patterns. If there were doubts about a diagnosis when someone was

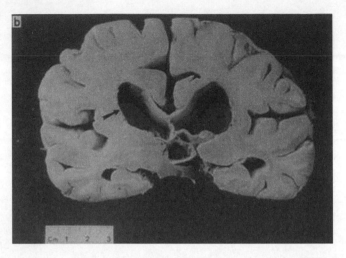

Figure 9.3 Photograph of a cut brain from someone with Huntington's disease. Both the cortex and the basal ganglia are damaged but it is clear that the brunt of the damage occurs in the basal ganglia. This figure was published in Huntington's Diesease, Ed Harper PS, 1991, page 145. Copyright Elsevier.

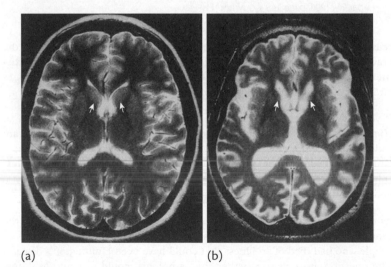

(a)   (b)

Figure 9.4 Pictures of brain scans from someone without Huntington's disease (a) and with Huntington's disease (b), in which the loss of nerve cells in the area of the basal ganglia can be seen.

alive, then it was very helpful if a pathologist reported that the pattern of change in the brain was typical of Huntington's disease.

Are other areas of the brain affected?

The answer to this is 'yes'. Although the brunt of the damage occurs to the basal ganglia, subtle changes occur to other areas of the brain. These can be seen with the help of a microscope, but need not be considered in detail in this book. Instead, I want to say more about the basal ganglia.

What is the function of the basal ganglia?

If the basal ganglia are badly damaged in Huntington's disease, then it is reasonable to ask what functions the basal ganglia normally control and how the damage relates to the clinical features, which were described in Chapters 2, 3, and 4. At a very simple level we could suggest that the nerve cells in the basal ganglia are involved in co-ordinating activities in the cortex to signal changes in various muscles to give a smooth pattern of movements. A computer can be used to program a robot, but the movements are step-wise and jerky, as opposed to the smooth movements we use. A sequence of movements can be learnt: if you get up to go to the door, complex changes in the muscles can be co-ordinated without you thinking about the individual steps. A similar co-ordinating role probably applies to give a smooth sequence of thoughts. The next question is, 'How?'

Although this is far from clear, we have an understanding of a series of connections between the cortex and the basal ganglia, which can be likened to a wiring diagram. In fact, two pathways can be recognized: the first is the **indirect pathway** (Fig. 9.5a) and the second is the **direct** pathway (Fig. 9.5b). Both pathways from the basal ganglia are damaged in Huntington's disease.

The output of a nerve cell can either **excite** or **inhibit** the next nerve cell in the pathway. If a nerve cell is excited it will send more messages to the next nerve cell; conversely, if it is inhibited it will send fewer. The combination of inhibitory and excitatory signals in the pathways is confusing. The motor cortex sends excitatory signals to the basal ganglia, but if these cells are damaged the balance of the direct and indirect pathways back to the cortex is altered, resulting in a movement disorder. This is the key point, but we can consider the pathways in more detail. In broad terms, damage to the indirect pathway tends to produce **chorea**, whereas damage to the direct pathway tends to produce slowness of movement or **bradykinesia**. As we saw in Chapter 2, chorea is an early sign of Huntington's disease so we would expect the indirect pathway to be relatively more vulnerable in the early stages of the disease.

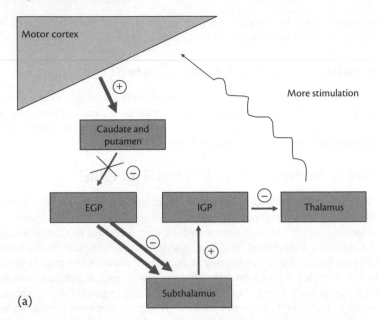

Figure 9.5 (a) Diagram of the indirect pathway. The caudate and putamen parts of the basal ganglia are damaged in Huntington's disease. For the indirect pathway, this involves loss of inhibitory impulses to the external globus pallidus (EGP), shown by the crossed-out arrow. This means that there is much more inhibition of the subthalamus. This leads to less stimulation of the internal globus pallidus (IGP) and less inhibition of the thalamus, which in turn means more stimulation back to the cortex. – indicates inhibitory signals, + indicates excitatory signals.

The indirect pathway is shown in Figure 9.5a. It involves an area of the brain called the **subthalamus**. In other situations, damage to the subthalamus results in extra movements. If we go through the indirect pathway carefully, we can work out that damage to the caudate/putamen results in increased neurochemical inhibition of the subthalamus. The cortex sends stimulatory signals to the caudate/putamen, which should send inhibitory signals to the **external globus pallidus** which, in turn, should send inhibitory signals to the subthalamus. Damage to the caudate/putamen results in less inhibition of the external globus pallidus. This, in turn, results in increased inhibition of the subthalamus. The effect of increased inhibition of the subthalamus is that there is less stimulation of the **internal globus pallidus,** which in turn leads to less inhibition of the **thalamus** and more stimulation from the thalamus to the cortex. The net effect is over-activity of movement.

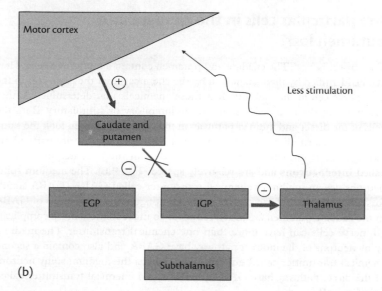

Figure 9.5 (b) Diagram of the direct pathway. Loss of the direct pathway from damage to the caudate and putamen in Huntington's disease means there is less inhibition of the internal globus pallidus (IGP), shown by the crossed-out arrow, and therefore more inhibition of the thalamus and less stimulation back to the cortex. – indicates inhibitory signals, + indicates excitatory signals.

Damage to the direct pathway is easier to follow because there are fewer steps. The cortex sends stimulatory signals to the caudate/putamen, which should send inhibitory signals to the **internal globus pallidus**. This step in the pathway is damaged, so there is increased inhibition of the thalamus and less stimulation from the thalamus back to the cortex and under-activity of movement.

Although it is confusing, the fact that there are two pathways helps explain why we see a mixture of movement disorders in Huntington's disease. Disturbance of the balance between these pathways results in chorea, which is often seen early in the course of the disease. However, as the disease progress further, disturbance to the balance of the indirect and direct pathways results in slow movements and dystonic postures (as described in Chapter 2). This explanation goes a long way to explain the neurological signs seen in Huntington's disease, but it does not quite explain them all so further refinement can be expected in the future.

Are particular cells in the caudate and putamen lost?

The answer is 'yes'. The caudate and putamen contain a mixture of cells. They can be identified by their shape and by the chemicals that they transmit to the next nerve cell in the pathway. It is these chemicals that determine whether the effect on the next cell is going to be inhibitory or stimulatory. Both the cells of the direct and indirect pathway in the caudate/putamen look the same and are called **medium spiny neurons**. It is these cells that are particularly damaged in Huntington's disease. Other cells in the caudate/putamen are called **interneurons** and are relatively spared (Fig. 9.6). The medium spiny neurons use an inhibitory chemical transmitter called GABA (GABA stands for 'gamma-aminobutyric acid'), and in Huntington's disease levels of GABA in the caudate/putamen are much reduced. To make matters more complicated, nerve cells can have more than one chemical transmitter. The medium spiny neurons of the indirect pathway have GABA and also contain a second chemical transmitter called **enkephalin**, whereas the medium spiny neurons of the direct pathway have GABA plus a second chemical transmitter called **substance P**.

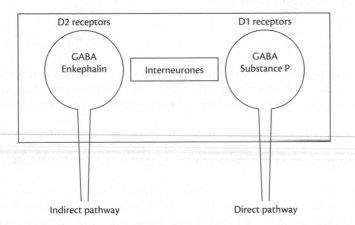

Figure 9.6 Diagram to show the different nerve cell types in the caudate and putamen. Those medium spiny neurons that contain GABA and enkephalin or GABA and substance P are particularly susceptible to loss in Huntington's disease. The interneurones, which use other chemical neurotransmitters, are relatively spared.

Why do we treat with dopa blockers?

All neurons have receptors to receive signals or chemicals transmitted from other neurons. The medium spiny neurons have receptors for **glutamate** to receive the stimulatory signals from the cortex. They also have receptors for another chemical called **dopamine** or 'dopa'. There are two categories of dopamine receptor: D1 and D2. In general terms, the D2 receptors are on the medium spiny neurons of the indirect pathway and the D1 receptors are on the medium spiny neurons of the direct pathway. The D2 receptors inhibit the medium spiny neurons of the indirect pathway when a dopamine molecule attaches to them. Generally speaking, there is a relative excess of dopamine compared with other parts of the brain. Inhibition of these neurons cumulatively adds to the fact that they are damaged and contributes to the chorea. This can be treated by using a drug that depletes the amount of dopamine present or, alternatively, blocks the dopamine receptors. Treatment with these drugs, known as dopamine or dopa blockers, will alter the balance of the indirect and direct pathways such that chorea is reduced and slowness of movement or bradykinesia increased, but it will not slow down the progressive damage that occurs in Huntington's disease.

Can the changes in the brain explain some of the personality changes?

The question of understanding some of the personality changes has been difficult because of confounding issues, such as depression, and the fact that the cortex is affected to some extent as well as the basal ganglia. Broadly speaking, doctors classify dementia as **cortical** or **subcortical**. Alzheimer's disease falls into the cortical dementia category, because the cortex is where most of the damage occurs. Huntington's disease, Parkinson's disease, and a few other rare disorders are considered to be subcortical dementias. This terminology clearly describes the fact that the basal ganglia are below the cortex. As a broad generalization, people with subcortical dementia have slowed thinking and learning, but, unlike those with cortical dementia, have not lost the ability to comprehend.

Neuropsychologists are scientists who specialize in testing specific thinking processes. We are all familiar with the idea of an IQ test. In fact, this is not one test but is composed of several tests. In addition to IQ, there are many tests that try to assess different intellectual processes. In a clinic, a medical doctor may use very simple tests, including asking the precise date, asking about the precise location, asking for three words to be learnt, and copying a diagram. You may have come across these if you have attended a clinic with a relative who is affected. The advantage of a test like this is that it is quick and simple, but more detailed tests require a lot more time to complete.

The movement disorder can result from a disturbance of the circuit from the motor cortex through the basal ganglia (caudate/putamen). Similarly, the problems with thinking and behaviour result from disturbance of circuits from the frontal cortex through the basal ganglia (caudate/putamen). There are similarities between patients with Huntington's disease and those who have damage to the frontal cortex. In general terms these result in damage to **executive function**. This implies problems with planning ahead, switching between tasks, and the flexibility to make changes in response to new information. The net effect is an increase in apathy and more irritability.

➡ Summary

We can summarize some of the key messages about changes in the brain from this section:

◆ Loss of nerve cells is selective.

◆ Several areas of the brain are damaged but the brunt of the damage is in two areas called the caudate and putamen nuclei.

◆ Cells in the caudate and putamen that contain GABA are particularly sensitive to the damage caused by Huntington's disease. These cells are called medium spiny neurons.

◆ There are two types of medium spiny neurone and two types of pathway from the caudate/putamen: the indirect and direct pathways. Both pathways are damaged in Huntington's disease.

◆ There is some explanation for the movement disorder seen in Huntington's disease.

◆ Current treatments can reduce chorea but not slow down the progressive nerve cell damage.

◆ How the damage leads to abnormal thought processes is less clearly understood.

10

What causes selective nerve cell damage?

> ## ➡ Key points
>
> ◆ The cause of the selective nerve cell damage is unknown.
>
> ◆ Abnormal huntingtin is found in both affected and unaffected cells.
>
> ◆ Normal and abnormal huntingtin have many functions in cells.
>
> ◆ A hallmark of Huntington's disease is that the first part of the protein is cut, and the small fragment forms aggregates that are not cleared by the cell.
>
> ◆ The role of the aggregates is unclear.
>
> ◆ Current experiments probably study the later stages of nerve cell damage, whereas we need to understand what triggers the damage to some nerve cells and the early steps in the process.

This chapter focuses on ideas and research activity to explain why specific nerve cells die in Huntington's disease. A problem in writing this chapter is that we do not yet have a complete explanation. This means that there are various loose ends. Understanding the detail of how the abnormal huntingtin protein results in a specific pattern of cell death is more than an academic exercise; it is essential to the development of treatments that will prevent or significantly delay the cell death in those at risk. I will start with ideas that were being developed before the gene was cloned. I will then go on to explain why there is still difficulty in understanding the step from an abnormal huntingtin protein to nerve cells that are sick and then to nerve cells that die.

Are the nerve cells being murdered or do they commit suicide?

This is a dramatic way of expressing the problem. Alternatively, you could ask if the gene for Huntington's disease produces a toxic substance that kills these cells, or if there is something about these cells in Huntington's disease that means that they are programmed to die back prematurely. In order to think about this we need to consider an animal model.

Why do we need an animal model?

An animal model allows experiments to be undertaken to answer questions about the basic problem that causes Huntington's disease. Whilst this is important, an animal model would also allow treatment options to be considered and worked out. Clearly, if a treatment slowed down the disease process in an animal model then it would be worth trying on people affected by Huntington's disease. Unfortunately, there are no animals that naturally develop a similar disorder. This means that the disease has to be induced in the animal models that are available.

Are there chemicals that cause damage similar to Huntington's disease?

The answer to this is 'yes'. One of the chemical messengers between nerve cells is glutamate. Experiments in 1969 showed that if a nerve cell receives too much stimulation from glutamate then it will die. As we saw in the last chapter, glutamate is the chemical messenger between the cortex of the brain and the basal ganglia. One model of Huntington's disease is to inject glutamate, or chemicals similar to glutamate, into the basal ganglia of a rat or a monkey and see which nerve cells are most vulnerable to the effects of the toxin. This model produces results that are surprisingly similar to the damage caused by Huntington's disease in humans. These experiments have been refined over the years so that chemicals which produce a near perfect match with Huntington's disease have been identified.

As we saw in the last chapter, chemical messengers cross the gap between nerve cells. The chemical message is detected by receptors on the surface of the next nerve cell. Specific chemical messengers are detected by specific receptors. Some experiments identified that chemicals which mimicked the damage caused by Huntington's disease used a subgroup of the glutamate receptors called NMDA receptors. These are named after one of the chemicals that cause their stimulation.

This type of model has been very useful in helping to define which cells in the basal ganglia are especially damaged by Huntington's disease and which are relatively spared; it also suggests that the NMDA receptor is involved in the disease process. The model was developed in the 1980s before anything was known about the nature of the expansion of part of the gene or the abnormal protein huntingtin. In this model the nerve cells are being 'murdered' by a toxic substance.

More recent modifications to the model

Huntington's disease does not usually develop until adulthood and is slowly progressive for many years. This is completely different from what happens when we inject a toxic substance into the brain of an animal, which produces immediate damage. There are other problems with the model, including the fact that high levels of a toxic substance are not found in the brains of people with Huntington's disease. In the early 1990s a modification to the model was proposed.

There is evidence for abnormal energy levels in some of the cells in the brain. We know that we eat sugar (glucose) to obtain energy. The sugar is converted to energy in parts of the cell called **mitochondria**. It is possible to inject a chemical into the bodies (*not* the brains) of laboratory animals that damages the energy production in the mitochondria. This results in a slower effect on the brain and results in a strikingly similar pattern of nerve cell damage. In patients with Huntington's disease it is possible to perform specialized brain scans that show changes in energy production in the brain. Perhaps the abnormal energy production in the cells increases the susceptibility of the NMDA receptor to toxic damage from glutamate.

These ideas were also being developed at a time before the abnormality in the gene was known. It would have been marvellous if the discovery of the gene and the way in which the huntingtin protein is abnormal had explained why some cells are damaged. Unfortunately, this has not proved to be the case.

The nature of the problem

It is often said that we have about 30,000 genes. There are a very large number of genetic conditions and many of the mistakes or mutations that cause them have been discovered in recent years. It would be tempting to think that there

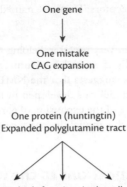

One gene

↓

One mistake
CAG expansion

↓

One protein (huntingtin)
Expanded polyglutamine tract

Multiple functions in the cell

Figure 10.1 Diagram showing the basic understanding of the changes in Huntington's disease. Our problem with understanding the basic cause is that both the normal and abnormal huntingtin have multiple functions within cells.

is one gene for each genetic disease. This is frequently not the case: sometimes, the same genetic disease can result from different mistakes in one or more genes. To make matters more complex, sometimes different genetic diseases can result from mistakes in the same gene. In Huntington's disease the situation appears to be more simple: we have seen that there is one mistake in one gene, which makes one protein (Fig. 10.1). So why do we not understand why this one abnormal protein causes damage to the cell? One reason for this is that huntingtin is involved in a number of different cellular processes, and so the abnormal huntingtin damages a number of different cellular processes. As yet it is not possible to understand how these abnormal processes link together to cause selective nerve cell damage. I find it helpful to describe this as having 'islands of knowledge'.

What were some of the first questions asked when huntingtin was identified?

One way of trying to determine the function of huntingtin was to see if it was similar to any other protein that had been identified. This was done, and it was quickly realized that huntingtin was not similar to any protein whose function was already known.

In Chapter 5 we noted that genes are present in every cell but that in any particular cell most of the genes are inactive. The converse of this is that in any particular cell or tissue only some genes are actively expressing their protein product. Since some cells are selectively damaged in Huntington's disease, it is reasonable to ask if huntingtin is selectively expressed in these cells. Again, it was soon realized that huntingtin was widely expressed in all tissues but, more importantly, was present in all nerve cells. In brain tissue from patients with Huntington's disease both the normal and abnormal protein were expressed. These results were disappointing because they gave no clue to the underlying cause of the cell death in Huntington's disease. The fact that abnormal huntingtin is widely expressed means that just having a longer polyglutamine tract does not, by itself, cause nerve cell death.

Another approach to the problem was to see if huntingtin was localized to a specific part of the cell. Figure 10.2 is a diagram showing the normal localization of huntingtin. Although some of the early results were contradictory, most studies indicated that huntingtin was not in the nucleus (which contains the genetic material). Normal huntingtin is mostly found outside the nucleus, in the **cytoplasm**. Although this was progress, it still did not answer some of the basic questions about the cause of the selective cell death in Huntington's disease.

A different approach was, and still is, to identify other proteins that interact with huntingtin. Normal-sized huntingtin must interact with other proteins to produce a normal function. In the case of Huntington's disease the larger huntingtin protein must gain a new function and this somehow leads to selective nerve cell death. Since the gene has been identified, huntingtin has been found to interact with a number of other proteins. The function of some of these proteins is known but some of the other proteins have not been previously recognized. I have chosen not to list the various proteins with which huntingtin interacts because it is still not clear from this work how having the abnormal huntingtin leads to the selective nerve cell death typical of Huntington's disease.

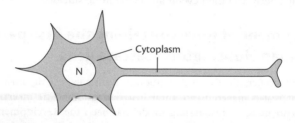

Figure 10.2 Diagram showing the main position of huntingtin outside the nucleus (**N**).

Gain of function or loss of function?

A mistake or mutation in a gene may result in the protein it produces being damaged, so that the protein it is *supposed* to produce is not present or does not function properly. Scientists describe this as a **loss of function mutation**. Alternatively, a mistake or mutation could result in the gene producing a protein that does something new within the cell which causes damage. This is called a **gain of function mutation**. Before the gene was discovered there was evidence to suggest that the problem in Huntington's disease was a gain of function mutation. This would make sense, as the abnormal polyglutamine tract in the huntingtin protein would alter its shape and result in it doing something new within the cell to cause problems. We have to be open to the idea that if huntingtin has a number of different functions, the problems with the cell could be a mixture of loss of a normal function and gain of a new function.

This idea of a gain of function was supported by a series of studies that were done soon after the gene was discovered. It is possible to breed mice with one damaged copy of the gene and see what happens. In this type of experiment some mice ought to be born with *both* copies of the gene damaged. The interesting result was that these mice were not born but died before birth. The conclusion from this series of experiments is that huntingtin is important for normal development. Of course this is the wrong model; we need mice or laboratory animals that produce an abnormal protein. There are no animals that develop Huntington's disease in nature, so the abnormal gene needs to be inserted into animals to model the disease.

As cells age, they die. If they died by bursting open, then the contents of the cell would damage the surrounding tissue, which would become inflamed. In order to avoid this, cells have a mechanism to quietly 'commit suicide' without causing further damage. This mechanism is sometimes called **programmed cell death** and occurs in many tissues of the body. It is reasonable to ask if the gain of function mutation in the Huntington gene results in some cells functioning poorly and then eventually committing suicide.

Development of mice containing the first part of the human Huntington's disease gene

It is possible to genetically modify laboratory animals, usually mice, so that a gene of interest is inserted into their genetic material. The inserted gene is called a **transgene**. A fascinating model has been the development of mice that have been genetically modified to contain the first part of the human

Huntington's disease gene. Mice with this type of modification are called **transgenic**. The mice containing the first part of the gene had a very large polyglutamine expansion. A mouse does not live as long as a human, so very large expansions were chosen (similar to those seen in juvenile Huntington's disease) in order that the disease process was amplified and changes could be seen during the lifetime of the mouse.

In these mice abnormal movements and neurological signs were present. These abnormal neurological signs were not entirely typical of Huntington's disease, but we have to remember these were genetically modified mice, not humans. At first, examination of the brains of the transgenic mice was disappointing: they were smaller than normal mouse brains, but otherwise not especially remarkable.

In 1997, detailed studies of the nerve cells of these mice showed that they contained clumps or aggregates of protein material in the **nucleus** of the cell. As you will recall, this is not a part of the cell that normally contains huntingtin. These clumps of protein contain the first part of the protein. Once this discovery had been made, it was soon realized that these clumps had first been seen in electron microscopic studies in 1979 but no-one had realized their significance. Since this discovery, the brains of patients with Huntington's disease have been re-examined and the same clumps have been found in the cortex and basal ganglia.

Do the aggregates contain huntingtin?

In order to answer this question we have to consider the technical aspect of how huntingtin is detected in a cell. The process involves raising an **antibody** to huntingtin. We now have to consider what an antibody is. When children are vaccinated, a doctor or nurse injects proteins from a bacteria or virus into them. The children's immune system recognizes these proteins as foreign and produces antibodies specific to them. When the children encounter the live bacteria or virus, their immune system immediately recognizes the foreign proteins and can now rapidly produce more relevant antibodies. The antibodies bind to the bacteria or virus, which makes it easier for the immune system to destroy them. A vaccination programme prevents the vast majority of children from developing specific infections.

Once huntingtin was identified, antibodies were raised to the protein so that it could be detected in various parts of the cell. Interestingly, the aggregates were only detected when antibodies to the first part of the protein were used. This implies that the large huntingtin protein is cut within the cell. This cutting of a large protein is a normal process within a cell.

A small protein that contains a large stretch of glutamines will tend to form clumps, as shown in Figure 10.3. The huntingtin protein is actually very large and is normally located outside the nucleus. As part of the normal process in the cell, the huntingtin protein is cut. If the first part contains a normal stretch of glutamines then the cell works normally, but if it contains a large stretch of glutamines then it will form aggregates. These aggregates can form in the nucleus, the cell body, and the dendrites or projections and axon. Another protein is found in the aggregates, called **ubiquitin**. A protein labelled with ubiquitin is normally a mechanism for indicating that the cell should get rid of that protein. The fact that clumps form may mean that the pathway for getting rid of the protein is overwhelmed.

In the experimental mice the aggregates form and the mice show abnormal behaviours before the nerve cells die. In fact the mice die before there are major changes in the brain. This suggests that a lot of the problems seen in Huntington's are due to cells being sick and functioning poorly, with cell death occurring at a later stage.

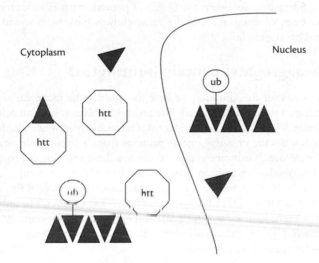

Figure 10.3 Diagram showing that the huntingtin protein (**htt**) is cut. The abnormally large first part of the protein with the expanded polyglutamine tract (represented by the triangle) forms clumps both inside and outside the nucleus. The clumps are bound to the protein ubiquitin (**ub**), which marks proteins for clearance. The clumps are not cleared by the cell. Other important proteins can be caught in the clumps.

As the aggregates form, other proteins get caught in the process, so the reduction of these proteins in the cell might account for some of the problems that are seen. Some of the proteins that get caught in the aggregates in the nucleus may be important for controlling the function of other genes. Getting these proteins trapped may be a mechanism for explaining some of the problems that occur in the cell.

Are aggregates good, bad, or indifferent?

At first sight, this seems a curious question. Aggregates are now recognized as a hallmark of Huntington's disease. The problem again is that this represents an island of knowledge. There is no formal proof that aggregates are the main cause of cells becoming sick. If aggregates are bad for the cell, then looking for drugs that reduce the number of aggregates should help. On the other hand, it could be that the aggregates are a mechanism by which the cell is trying to protect itself from a gain of function of the abnormal huntingtin protein. If this is the case, then drugs that increase aggregation would be helpful. A third possibility is that the aggregates are an unimportant side issue and unrelated to the main damage to the cell. Intuitively, aggregates seem to be a bad thing, but until we are able to tell a complete story it is important to keep an open mind.

Are aggregates seen in other disorders?

The answer to this is 'yes'. Huntington's disease is not the only disorder to be characterized by an expansion of a polyglutamine repeat. A few other neurological disorders are caused by exactly the same mechanism, although the proteins involved are different from huntingtin. These other neurological disorders are also characterized by selective nerve cell death but the pattern is specific for each of them. The discovery of aggregates in Huntington's disease prompted similar studies to be undertaken in brains of patients with these disorders, and sure enough aggregates have been found. This must be telling us something: the expansion of the polyglutamine repeat by itself does not cause selective nerve cell damage. The expansions occur within specific proteins, and it is the expansion within the particular protein that causes a specific pattern of nerve cell damage which is characteristic for each of these diseases.

What about other models?

Various models have been devised. In one, the full length of the protein is put into a mouse so that the stages of cutting the huntingtin protein can be studied.

Perhaps a more accurate model is to increase the length of the CAG repeat sequence (which codes for the polyglutamine stretch) in the normal mouse gene. Models have been made with fruit flies and cells. Having got a cellular or animal model of Huntington's disease, it is possible to think about treating the cells or animals with drugs to reverse the damage. To date, this has not resulted in the development of new drugs to try out on patients, but I will come back to this point in the next chapter.

Blind men studying an elephant

This chapter described two different ways to explain the selective nerve cell death. Neither explanation is complete in itself. Although it is not possible to provide a detailed explanation of the cause of the selective nerve cell death, considerable progress in understanding has occurred in the last few years.

In one explanation, the abnormal huntingtin somehow leads to abnormal energy production of some cells, which renders them more vulnerable to the toxic effects of chemical messengers in the brain. How the abnormal huntingtin leads to abnormal energy production is unclear.

In the other explanation, the large huntingtin protein is cut. If the first part contains a large expansion of glutamines then it forms clumps and is labelled with ubiquitin but not cleared from the cell. It may be the case that this interferes with a number of different pathways in the cell and that a later stage in the process is a problem with energy production. There are still a lot of unanswered questions, including an explanation for the selective cell death seen in Huntington's disease.

If blind men study an elephant they will come to different conclusions: some men will feel the trunk, others will study the feet, and others still will study the tail. There seems to be a similar issue in Huntington's disease. The protein with the expanded polyglutamine stretch is a problem within the cell. Something triggers an abnormal process in the cell such that a number of different events take place, some of which ultimately lead to cells being sick and then dying (Fig. 10.4). Different groups of scientists are studying these abnormal processes but as yet no-one is able to stand back and piece them together into a coherent story. Ideally, the factors that trigger an abnormal response and the very early steps of the cell becoming sick need to be identified.

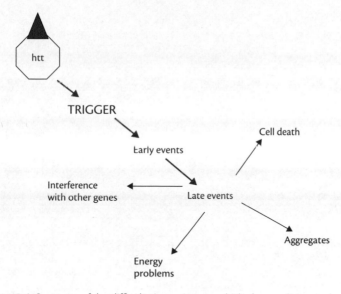

Figure 10.4 Summary of the difficulty in sorting out which abnormalities are the primary cause of poorly functioning cells and ultimately selective cell death.

Conclusion

It is disappointing that the mechanism that causes the specific pattern of nerve cell damage remains unclear. A lot of research work has focused on the role of the aggregates that occur in the cells. Clearly, they have to be explained, and in the next chapter I will go on to describe future research strategies that involve both clinics and basic research scientists.

11

Current research activities

> ## ➡ Key points
>
> ◆ Scientists and clinicians interested in Huntington's disease have organized large research networks.
>
> ◆ Suggested treatments need to be assessed in large clinical trials and the infrastructure for this is now in place.
>
> ◆ Methods to improve the way we decide whether a treatment is effective are being developed.
>
> ◆ Research is focusing on the early changes that occur in Huntington's disease.
>
> ◆ Work is continuing on developing nerve cell transplants.

In the last chapter, I discussed research activities based in laboratories that focus on animal models and studies of cells. In this chapter, I would like to consider research activities that involve patients and families. I do not want to be too optimistic that effective treatment is around the corner and that all will be well in a few years' time. Of course, I would be delighted if this were to be the case. On the other hand, if Huntington's disease affects you or your relatives, it is important that ideas for effective treatment are being considered and that the research activity I have described in the previous chapter is leading somewhere.

I also want to emphasize that there is a difference between an effective treatment and a cure. If someone has a serious infection and is treated with appropriate antibiotics, then the person can be restored to good health and cured. On the other hand, if someone has a chronic condition like diabetes, then giving them insulin is a very effective treatment, but the injections with insulin do not cure the underlying damage, which in this example is to cells in the pancreas.

Formation of networks

In Chapters 2, 3, and 4, I was careful not to name any specific drugs, but rather mentioned the main classes of drugs that are currently used to treat Huntington's disease. This is because I do not want to give the impression that one particular drug is better than another. In order to assess whether a drug is effective, a clinical trial is undertaken. For many of the drugs that are used to treat Huntington's disease, the trials were done some years ago and involved small numbers of patients. In assessing whether a drug is effective, there has to be an outcome which is measured. One obvious outcome to measure is a reduction in the abnormal movements. For a lot of studies this was the main outcome which was assessed. Unfortunately, Huntington's disease is more complex than this, and it might be better to have a range of outcomes to measure. A group of researchers have devised a scale that assesses movements, thinking and behaviour, and functional capacity (the ability to undertake a variety of tasks, such as going to work, driving, shopping, washing, and dressing) called the Unified Huntington's Disease Rating Scale, or UHDRS. This rating scale can assess the rate of progression of Huntington's disease and is used to assess treatments.

In order to assess treatments, large numbers of patients are needed and a large number of doctors and other researchers need to make the assessments. This requires a period of training for those doctors and researchers to make sure that they all assess the patients in the same way.

One response to this problem has been the development of research networks. The research network in North America was developed first and is called the Huntington Study Group or HSG. More recently, a similar network has been developed in Europe called the European Huntington's Disease Network or EHDN. This allows details from a large group of patients to be assembled together, clinical assessments to be made, and samples of blood and urine to be collected. Having gathered these resources together, a number of studies can be undertaken, as shown in the summary.

➜ Summary of the activities of research networks

- ◆ Improving the effectiveness of the current rating scales.

- ◆ Developing new markers for the disease.

- ◆ Identifying the very earliest changes in Huntington's disease.

- ◆ Undertaking clinical trials of drugs.

Why improve the current rating scales?

There is no ideal way of assessing the abilities of someone with Huntington's disease so a variety of different assessments are used and represent a compromise. An ideal rating scale should be objective so that, no matter which doctor or researcher assesses the patient, they all give the same answer. Moreover, having a standardized way of assessing patients means that researchers can compare results between different studies and all be aware of the strengths and weaknesses of the different parts of the rating scales.

You can imagine the problem if I tell you that one of the assessments is how much chorea is present in the left hand and that the score can be 0, 1, 2, 3 or 4 (with '0' being 'no chorea', and '4' being 'severe chorea'). Different researchers might have different ideas of what is minimal, mild, moderate or severe chorea. Their objectivity can be improved by training days so that they agree on what is meant and by giving researchers written descriptions of each category to guide them.

In an earlier part of the book, I explained that a person can be affected with Huntington's disease for a long time and that the features of Huntington's disease can vary over time. A rating scale may thus be very helpful for most patients, but may be less helpful in the very early or the very late stages, or indeed if the age of onset is young. There is therefore scope to refine and improve the current methods of assessment. We also need to define more clearly what is meant by an improvement. Controlling the chorea may sometimes be helpful, but a better measure of outcome may be an improvement in thinking or in mood. A measure called a 'quality of life' measure may also be used to assess how someone's well-being has changed, rather than measuring a change in a symptom of Huntington's disease. This approach recognizes that the symptoms of Huntington's disease may not affect everyone in the same way.

Why do we want a new marker when we have the DNA test?

The answer to this question is best illustrated by Figure 11.1. If someone has inherited the gene for Huntington's disease, the result of the genetic test will be the same at conception, at birth, when the person is a child, when the person is an adult and has no signs of the condition, and when the person is in the early, middle, and late stages of the disease. The result of the genetic test is valuable, but it does not help with assessing the stage of the condition. As you can see from Figure 11.1, we think there has been a lot of damage to the nerve cells before a doctor makes a clinical diagnosis. If we had a test on blood or

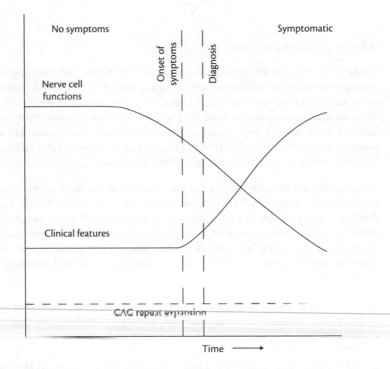

Figure 11.1 Timeline of Huntington's disease. The dotted line represents the results of the genetic test, which remains the same during both the preclinical and symptomatic stages. The upper solid line represents changes in nerve cell function, which start to be abnormal before the onset of problems. The lower solid line represents changes in clinical features, which can be observed by families and doctors. The gap between the two vertical lines indicates the period between someone starting with symptoms and at a later time a diagnosis being made. (Based on slide from Dr Tabrizi).

urine that varied between unaffected and affected people and between the different stages of the illness, then that would be of enormous help in assessing the effectiveness of any interventions.

In the previous section I described the fact that, despite training, there will always be some variability in the way different researchers assess patients. One way of minimizing this problem is to increase the number of patients in any particular study. This seems straightforward, but of course the need to assess large numbers of patients increases the financial cost of any study. If the assessments could be supplemented by another marker then that could reduce the number of patients who would need to participate in studies in order to give meaningful results.

What about the earliest changes?

A number of people have had predictive tests and know that they will develop Huntington's disease at some point in the future. If you look at Figure 11.1, you see there has been some damage to the nerve cells before a doctor can diagnose that Huntington's disease has started. If we could know more reliably what the very earliest changes are that occur in a person with Huntington's disease, then we would have a better understanding of the condition and ideally would want to target treatments at this stage. Anything that delays progression of the condition at this time would have an enormous benefit.

What about clinical trials?

Clinical trails have been undertaken in both Europe and North America. Assessing a pool of patients in detail has meant that the results have been obtained from a large group of patients in a much shorter time than was possible a few years ago. Developing a number of different cell lines and animal models into which the abnormal gene has been inserted means that a number of different possibilities can now be tried before going as far as a full trial in humans. We cannot know when an effective treatment will become available, but the current work means that we are better placed to assess current and future treatments. In the meantime, we have now got the mechanism to assess proposed new treatments in both the USA and Europe using efficient large-scale trials.

If you have participated in a clinical trial then you will know that it is a significant time commitment to attend extra clinics and have extra assessments. This is worthwhile, because we need to be sure that any treatments we recommend are based on evidence that they are helpful. Ideally, the results of a trial should clearly indicate whether a proposed treatment is, or is not, going to be helpful. It is disappointing if a proposed treatment does not show a significant benefit in a trial, but this information is definitely worth having. We have to arrange a trial when a treatment is first suggested. If a drug treatment is used without a full trial because of initial enthusiasm, it then becomes very difficult, if not impossible, to test out questions about the value of the drug at a later date.

What about other factors that modify the effect of the Huntington's disease gene?

We know that on average the larger the size of the expansion, the earlier the age of onset. However, this is an average, and as we saw on page 60 there is such a wide variation around the average that it cannot be used in clinical practice. The implication of this is that there must be other factors, both genetic and non-genetic, which influence aspects of Huntington's disease. This raises the question, 'Why is this likely to be helpful?' The answer is that if the other factors could be identified, particularly those that are associated with a later onset or slower course of the disease, then these factors could become targets for effective treatment. Looking for factors that have a small effect means taking samples of blood from a lot of people with Huntington's disease, and in addition a lot of clinical information is required to know whether they started early or late or had a lot of movement or a lot of depression.

What about nerve cell transplants?

At first glance this seems a very radical solution to the problem. The basic idea is to replace the damaged nerve cells. We all know that people who die in major accidents can be used as a source of transplant organs. This is a traumatic issue for those involved; however, the thought that a heart or kidney is helping someone else live a near-normal life may be a source of comfort. Unfortunately, brain cells from people killed in accidents are not suitable for transplants. The problem is that these nerve cells are mature, and if they are removed, then the long processes that connect them to the next nerve cell would be cut. This leads on to consideration of fetal cells, which are still developing. These cells are round rather than long in shape, and have the ability to develop the long nerve processes and form connections when transplanted. As you might expect, the technique has been shown to work in laboratory experiments. In addition, the treatment is used in some cases of Parkinson's disease.

The next question is whether it will work in patients with Huntington's disease. There are two main issues: first, whether it is safe, and secondly, whether it is effective in slowing down the disease process. A number of transplants have been undertaken, but at this time they are still the subject of an international research programme so it is difficult to comment on the long-term benefit.

There are clear ethical issues, because the source of the cells is fetal tissue from abortions. Steps can be taken to ensure that the clinical team asking if the cells may be donated is separate from those involved in the transplant, which makes it less likely that those involved feel under pressure from the doctors caring for someone with Huntington's disease. The cells have to be taken at a specific time during development and the nervous tissue needs careful dissection. Given the essential requirements, there is unlikely to be enough source material even if the technique is effective; therefore there is an urgent need to develop another source of stem cells. This approach would be used in the later stages of the disease. It may well have a role in the future, but the ideal should be to develop a medical treatment that has an effect in the very early stages of the disease, or, even better, a treatment that could be given in the period prior to the onset, as shown in Figure 11.1.

In what context is the research taking place?

One theme of this chapter, and the previous chapter, is that research is taking place in the context of international collaboration. Most scientific groups work in universities. Any group of scientists can choose to work on Huntington's disease; no-one is obliged to be part of a network, but the fact that a large number of researchers want to work in this way suggests that it could be an effective motor for more powerful projects. In the next chapter, I will comment on the patients' organizations. I have always been impressed by the close collaboration between the patients' organizations and the research community. The networks include members of the patients' organization, and, in my opinion, this is all to the good. It is essential that research work is supported by families affected by Huntington's disease and that researchers are also keen to address questions posed by the families themselves.

Conclusion

In one sense, it is disappointing that the mechanism for the selective cell damage and death is still unclear. A lot of research is still being undertaken and the fact that it is now organized into large networks means that the potential for co-operation and collaboration is much increased. The research is being undertaken at various levels involving basic scientists, clinical doctors, and patients' organizations. This is a considerable achievement in itself and should be a source of optimism for the future.

12

Useful resources and contacts

Professionals from the World Federation of Neurology Huntington's Disease Research Group (WFNHDRG) and members of patients' organizations in the International Huntington Association (IHA) meet together twice a year. This has become a regular fixture for the international exchange of information between those affected by Huntington's disease in their families and researchers studying the condition. It may be worthwhile to record how these two groups started.

A group of six doctors interested in Huntington's disease met in Montreal at a World Federation of Neurology, Neurogenetics and Neuro-ophthalmology Congress in 1967. They resolved to meet every two years, and subsequent meetings have been held at different venues around the world. This origin explains the rather long title of World Federation of Neurology Huntington's Disease Research Group.

The first international meeting of patients' organizations occurred in 1974, when representatives from Canada and the United Kingdom met at the annual meeting of the American Huntington's Disease Organization. The Dutch patients' organization was founded in April 1976 and Marjorie Guthrie, widow of Woodie Guthrie (see page 3) was an invited speaker. One year later the World Federation of Neurology Huntington's Disease Research Group were due to meet in Leiden, the Netherlands, and the organizers arranged for a meeting of international patients' societies to take place in the same building. At that time there were representatives from the USA, Canada, the UK, Australia, Belgium, and the Netherlands. Two years later the research group met in Oxford and the patients' organization again arranged to meet in the same place at the same time. It was at that meeting, in 1979, that the IHA was officially formed. At the time of writing, there has been greater integration of the two groups, with a meeting in the autumn of 2007 in Dresden, Germany.

Table 12.1 Some aims of most lay organizations

To disseminate information about Huntington's disease to family members via newsletters and pamphlets
To disseminate knowledge about Huntington's disease to local doctors, social workers and nursing homes
To arrange or facilitate meetings of local groups of family members
Raising funds to employ staff who will visit and support family members
Raising funds to foster research
Raising funds to provide financial help for the membership

What is the role of a patients' organization?

To some extent the role of patients' organizations varies from country to country and from organization to organization. Some of the aims of most organizations are summarized in Table 12.1.

Should you join a patients' organization?

It is obviously a personal decision whether you join a patients' organization. Some people like to join organizations, whereas others do not. Given that Huntington's disease is a rare disorder, some families benefit from knowing that they are not unique. Involvement can simply be at the level of reading a newsletter, whereas others want to meet other families, attend lectures on the subject, and help with the fund-raising. At the very least you should be aware of the existence of the organizations so that it is possible to make contact in the future. A list of international addresses is given in the Appendix.

Glossary

Affect: another term for a person's mood or emotional disposition.

Amniocentesis: the technique of removing fluid from around a baby at about the sixteenth week of pregnancy.

Antibody: a protein produced by the body in response to a foreign protein. The antibody binds to the foreign body and helps with its removal. Antibodies are also used in scientific experiments to bind to specific proteins.

Autosomal dominant inheritance: a mutation or mistake in the DNA on one of the autosomes that is passed down from one generation to the next. The mutation dominates over the normal copy of the gene on the other autosome and causes a disease or condition to develop.

Autosome: any one of chromosomes 1–22, that is any of the non-sex chromosomes.

Axon: the long process of a nerve that transmits the impulse to the next neuron.

Basal ganglia: the collection of nerve cells below the cortex of the brain. A number of different areas can be identified; those important to Huntington's disease include the caudate and putamen.

Bradykinesia: an abnormal slowness of movement.

Caudate: part of the basal ganglia that is especially affected by Huntigton's disease.

Chorea: random, purposeless involuntary movements.

Chorion biopsy: this involves taking a small piece of the placenta or afterbirth during a pregnancy. This contains fetal cells that can be used for prenatal diagnosis. It is also sometimes called chorionic villus sampling (CVS).

Chromosome: a structure in the nucleus of a cell that contains a tightly coiled linear thread of DNA. With the exception of eggs and sperm every cell has 46 chromosomes, which are in pairs. Eggs and sperm contain only one chromosome from each pair and have 23 chromosomes.

Cognition: the process involved in knowing and thinking but distinct from emotion.

Cognitive flexibility: the ability to adapt plans and concentrate on more than one task.

Cognitive impairment: a reduction in the ability to think.

Cortex, cortical: the outer layer, in this context the outer layer of nerve cells of the brain.

Cytoplasm: the area of the cell outside the nucleus.

Delusions: false beliefs that are inconsistent with someone's knowledge or experience. Religious beliefs are excluded.

Dementia: the loss of intellectual power, usually as a result of an illness.

Disinhibition: being unrestrained by the usual social constraints on behaviour. This could include anger, swearing or inappropriate sexual advances.

DNA: an abbreviation of deoxyribonucleic acid. This is the chemical structure of the genetic material. It contains four types of nucleic acid: adenine, thymine, cytosine, and guanine (A, T, C, and G). These form the letters of the genetic code.

Dystonia: prolonged contraction of muscles, which results in the limbs, neck or face adopting unusual positions.

Executive functions: those parts of the brain concerned with planning ahead and switching between tasks.

Expanded polyglutamine tract: the enlargement of the series of glutamine building blocks in the first part of the huntingtin protein.

GABA: one of the neurotransmitters in the nerve cells of the caudate and putamen basal ganglia. Nerve cells that use this neurotransmitter are particularly susceptible to Huntington's disease.

Glutamate: one of the neurotransmitters of the brain. In the context of Huntington's disease it is the neurotransmitter from nerve cells in the cortex to the caudate and putamen basal ganglia.

Glutamine: one of the building blocks of proteins. There is a series of glutamine building blocks in the first part of the huntingtin protein.

Histones: proteins around which the DNA molecule is wound to form a chromosome.

Huntingtin: the protein coded by the gene for Huntington's disease. The normal protein has a repeat series of less than 36 glutamines whereas abnormal huntingtin has more than 36 repeats of glutamine.

Linkage: two genes close together on the same chromosome so that they are very likely to be inherited together.

Mania: a recognized psychiatric condition in which a person is very energetic and often has grandiose ideas, such as having extreme wealth.

Marker: a variation in the DNA molecule close to a gene of interest, in this case Huntington's disease, such that the marker and the gene are usually inherited together.

Metabolism: the process of turning food into useful products for the body. In the context of Huntington's disease the word relates to the production of energy.

Mitochondria: specialized parts of the cell involved in the production of energy from fats and sugars.

Morbid jealousy: an unreasonable belief that a partner is being unfaithful.

Mutation: a change in the DNA molecule that results in a disease; in Huntington's disease the mutation is an unstable expansion of a trinucleotide repeat.

Nerve cell body: the part of the nerve cell that does not include the projections for receiving or transmitting impulses.

NMDA: a subclass of glutamate receptor thought to be involved in Huntington's disease. The abbreviation is for a chemical called N-methyl-D-aspartate.

Nucleus: specialized part of a cell, which contains the genetic material.

Penetrance (of a gene): the proportion of people with a gene for a particular disease who actually develop the condition. In the case of Huntington's disease this is almost 100 per cent.

Polyglutamine tract: a section of the first part of the huntingtin protein, which contains a repeated number of building blocks called glutamine.

Predictive test: a test undertaken on individuals at risk of Huntington's disease before the condition has started to see if they have inherited the gene.

Projection: the area of the nervous system to which impulses are transmitted from a particular group of nerve cells.

Putamen: part of the basal ganglia especially sensitive to Huntington's disease.

Rigidity: stiffness of movement.

Subcortical: a general term for the nerve cells in the brain that are below the cortex.

Transgene: the insertion of a gene of interest into another cell. If it is inserted into an egg cell that eventually becomes an animal, such as a laboratory mouse, then the animal is said to be **transgenic**.

Triplet: a three-letter code of the DNA molecule, which specifies one of the building blocks of a protein.

Ubiquitin: a protein involved in the clearance of other proteins from cells.

Unstable expansion of trinucleotide repeat: the nature of the mutation in Huntington's disease and several other disorders. It refers to the fact that the normal gene has a code for one of the building blocks (in the case of Huntington's disease the building block in question is glutamine), which is repeated a number of times. The abnormal gene has a much larger number of repeats. It is unstable because the number of repeats can vary when it is inherited by the next generation.

Appendix

Contact details for Huntington's disease organizations

Argentina

Huntington Disease Society of Argentina
Catamarca 19, Rufino (Santa Fé) CP 6100, Argentina
Tel: 54-3382-428 658
Email: huntington_ar@elistas.net
Website: http://www.huntingtonargentina.com.ar

Australia

Australian Huntington Disease Association
Suite B, 11 Aberdare Road, Nedlands, 6009 WA, Australia
Tel: 61-8-9346 7599; Fax: 61-8-9346 7597
Email: national@huntingtonsaustralia.asn.au
Website: http://www.huntingtonsaustralia.asn.au

Austria

Östereichische Huntington Hilfe
Sibeliusstrasze 9/3/35, 1100 Vienna, Austria
Tel: 43-1-6150 265
Email:shg-huntington-wien@gmx.at
Website: http://www.huntington.at

Belgium (Flanders)

Huntington Liga

Krijkelberg 1, B 3360 Bierbeek, Belgium

Tel: 32-16-452 759; Fax: 32-16-452 760

Email: socialedienst@huntingtonliga.be

Website: http://www.huntingtonliga.be

Belgium (Wallonia)

Ligue Huntington Francophone Belge

4B Montagne Ste Walburge, 4000 Liege, Belgium

Tel: 32-4-225 8733; Fax: 32-4-225 8469

Email: info@huntington.be

Website: http://www.huntington.be

Brazil

Associacao Brasil Huntington

Rua Treze De Maio; 226 Centro, CEP 12940.720

Atibaia—Sao Paulo, Brasil

Tel/Fax: 55-11-4412 2199

Email: info@abh.org.br

Website: http://www.abh.org.br

Uniao dos Parentes e Amigos dos Doentes de Huntington

QE 32 Conjuno N Casa 25 Guara II

Brasilia—DF 71065-141, Brasil

Tel/Fax: 55 61 3036 1504

Email: contato@upadh.org.br

Website: http://www.upadh.org.br

Canada

Huntington Society of Canada

151 Frederick Street, Suite 400, N2H 2M2 Kitchener, Ontario, Canada

Tel: 1-519-749 7063; Fax: 1-519-749 8965

Email: info@huntingtonsociety.ca

Website: http://www.huntingtonsociety.org

Société Huntington du Quebec

2300 Boulevard René Lévesque O

Montréal, Quebec H3H 2R5, Canada

Tel: 1-514-282 4272; Fax: 1-514-937 0082

Email: shq@huntingtonqc.org

Website: http://www.huntingtonqc.ca

Colombia

Huntington Disease Society of Colombia

Calle 7#6-107, Juan de Acosta, Department of the Atlantic, Colombia

Email: fupehujac@hotmail.com

Cuba

Grupo Multidisciplinario para la Atención a Pacientes y Familiares con Diagnóstico de Enfermedad de Huntington

Instituto de Neurologia y Neurochirurgia

Dr Tatiana Zaldivar Vaillant

Calle 29 Esq D. Vedado

Havana City CP 10400, Cuba

Tel: 537-55 3034; Fax: 537-55 1820

Email: tzv@infomed.sld.cu

Czech Republic

Spolecnost pro Pomoc Pri Huntingtonove Chorobe

Velke Namesti 37

500 01 Hradec Kralove, Czech Republic

Tel/Fax: 420-491-421 334; Tel (home): 420-491-424 142

Email: info@huntington.cz

Website: http://www.huntington.cz

Denmark

Landsforeningen mod Huntington's Chorea

Falkoner Allé 80, 3. TV, 2000 Frederiksberg, Denmark

Tel: 45-9857 5323; Fax: 45-3536 0108

Email: sa.s@dadlnet.dk

Website: http://www.lhc.dk

Finland

Finnish Parkinson's Disease Association, Huntington Disease Branch

Rehabilitation Centre Suvituuli

Suvilinnantie 2, Postbox 905, 20100 Turku, Finland

Tel: 358-2-274 0412/358-2-5274 0421; Fax: 358-2-2740 444

Email: arja.pasila@parkinson.fi

Website: http://www.parkinson.fi

Finnish Huntington Association

Tuulensuunkatu 2, 20540 Turku, Finland

Tel: 358-2-237 4478

Email: heikki.tulento@fimnet.fi

France

Association Huntington France

42, 44 Rue du Chateau des Rentiers, 75013 Paris, France

Tel: 33-1-5360 0879; Fax: 33-1-5360 0899; Mobile: 06-7213 0958

Email: huntingtonfrance@wanadoo.fr

Website: http://huntington.fr

Fédération Huntington Espoir

20 Le Mas au Lièvre, BP26, F57645 Noisseville, France

Tel: 33-3-8776 6165; Fax: 33-3-8776 6165

Email: contact@huntington.asso.fr

Website: http://www.huntington.asso.fr

Germany

Deutsche Huntington Hilfe E.V.

Geschaefts- und Beratungsstelle

Boersenstrasse 10, D-47051 Duisburg, Germany

Tel: 49-203-22915; Fax: 49-203-22925,

Email: dhh@dhh-ev.de

Website: http://www.dhh-ev.de; www.selbsthilfenetz.de

Greece

Organization of Huntington in Greece

Hydras 13; 176-76 Athens, Greece

Tel: 1-951 8054; Mobile: 6973517827 or 6946161285

India

Huntington's Organization

P2-59 DLF Qutub Enclave Phase II, Gurgaon-122002 Haryana, India

Tel: 91-124-356 677; Fax: 91-124-351 945

Email: navnitsingh11@yahoo.com

Ireland

Huntington Disease Association of Ireland

Carmichael Centre, North Brunswick Street, Dublin 7, Ireland

Tel: 353-1-872 1303; Fax: 353-1-872 9931

Email:hdai@indigo.ie

Website: http://www.huntingtons.ie

Israel

Israeli Support Group for HD Families

3 Lubezky Street, Gedera 70700, Israel

Tel: 972-8-859 8573; Fax: 972-2-670 8387

Email: niradn@012.net.il

Italy

Associazione Italiana Corea di Huntington—Milano

C/O Fondazione IRCCS Istituto Neurologico "C. Besta"

Via Celoria 11, 20133 Milano, Italy

Tel: 39-02-239 4498; Fax: 39-02-2363 973

Email: info@aichmilano.it

Website: http://www.aichmilano.it

Associazione Italiana Corea di Huntington—Roma Onlus

Via Nomentana Nuova 56, 00161 Roma, Italy

Tel: 39-06-44292279/44242033; Fax: 39-06-44242033

Email: aich.roma@flashnet.it; info@aichroma.com

Website: http://www.aichroma.com

Associazione Italiana Corea di Huntington—Napoli

Policlinio Federico II, Clinica Neurologica—Ed 17

Via Pansini 5, 80131 Napoli, Italy

Tel: 39-081-5455 213; Fax: 39-081-7462 693

Email: aichnit@tin.it

Associazione Italiana Corea di Huntington—Neuromed

Via Atinense 18, 86077 Pozzilli (Is), Italy

Tel: 00390865-915238; 0039347-3132185; Fax: 00390865-927575

Email: levi@di.unipi.it; neurogen@neuromed.it

Website: http://www.di.unipi.it/~levi/sitoweb/index

Japan

Japanese Huntington's Disease Network

C/O Mrs Kaori Muto PhD

3-1-1 Asahi, Matsumoto, Nagano 390-8621, Japan

Tel/Fax: 81-263-37-2369

Email: jhdn@mbd.nifty.com

Website: http://www.jhdn.org

Malta

Huntington Self-Support Group Malta

Villa Aventura, Ant. Schembristreet

Sgn 06, Kappara, Malta G.C.

Tel: 356-9949 3267

Email:margaret@bridge.org.mt

Mexico

Asociacion Mexicana de la Enfermedad de Huntington I.A.P.

Tesorelos 97, Toriello Guerra Del. Tlalpan, 14050 Mexico City, Mexico

Tel: 52-5424 3325; Fax: 52-5424 3189

Email: asocia@prodigy.net.mx

The Netherlands

Vereniging van Huntington

Postbox 30470, 2500 Gl Den Haag, The Netherlands

Tel: 31-70-314 8888; Fax: 31-70-314 8880

Email: info@huntington.nl

Website: http://www.huntington.nl

New Zealand

Huntington's Disease Association (Wellington) New Zealand

4 Tainui Road

Titirangi, Auckland, New Zealand

Email: virginia.hogg@xtra.co.nz

Website: http://www.homepages.ihug.co.nz/~ghtaylor

Huntington's Disease Association (Canterbury) New Zealand

C/O Community House, 141 Hereford Street, Christchurch, Canterbury, New Zealand

Email: shirleyandbrian@paradise.net.nz

Northern Ireland

Huntington's Disease Association of Northern Ireland
8 Glenbank Close, Belfast BT17 0SN, Northern Ireland
Tel: 44-2890-221950
Email: s.mckay1@ntlworld.com
Website: http://www.northernirelandhd.tripod.com

Norway

Landsforeningen for Huntington's Sykdom
Tonstadbrinken 169, 7091 Tiller, Norway
Tel: 47-934-47795
Email: leder@huntington.no
Website: http://www.huntington.no

Pakistan

Huntington Disease Care and Cure Society of Pakistan
2 Sawati Gate, Peshawar Cantt, Pakistan
Tel: 92-091-275 471; Fax: 92-091-277 583
Email: hdccs@brain.net.pk

Pakistan Huntington Disease Society
Shifa Maternity Hospital
Zaryab Road, Zaryab Colony, Faqirabad No. 2
25000 Peshawar, Pakistan
Tel: 92-091-248747; Mobile: 92 03204951164
Email: dr_mussenmat@hotmail.com

Peru

Huntington Society of Peru (in establishment)
Mrs Maria Begazo Viza
Arequipa, Peru
Tel: 51-54-245 982; Fax: 51-54-211 1712
Email: mbegazo8@LatinMail.com

Poland

Stowarzyszenie na Rzecz Osób z Choroba Huntingtona w Polsce

Ogrodowa 9b/3 14-400 Paslek, Poland

Tel: 48-55-248 2044

Email: kontakt@huntington.pl

Website: http://www.huntington.pl

Portugal

Associacao Portuguesa de Doentes de Huntington

Rua Dr. Afonso Costa 32, L

P 8500-016 Alvor-Portimao, Portugal

Tel: 351-282-459 337; Fax: 351-282-459 337

Email: hd.ass.port@mail.telepac.pt

Website: http://www.apdh.4t.com

Russia

Huntington Association of Russia

Dr Sergey A. Klyushnikov

Institute of Neurology, Dept of Neurogenetics, Russian Academy of Medical Sciences

Volokolamskoye Shosse 80, 125367 Moscow, Russia

Tel: 7-95-490 2221; Fax: 7-95-490 2210

Email: sergeklyush@gmail.com; neurogen@online.ru

Slovakia

Spolecnost pre Pomoc pri Huntingtonovej Chorobe v Slovenskej Republike

Oddelinie Lekarskej Genetiky, 97517 Banska Bystrica, Slovakia

Tel: 42-88-713 380; Fax: 42-88-320 65

Email: mkva@grip.cis.upenn.edu

Slovenia

Huntington Association of Slovenia
Mr Rudolf Jakovac
Vrhovceva 13d, 1358 Log pri Brezovici
Tel: 386-1-7566 020; Fax: 386-1-560 3086
Email: ako9@siol.com

South Africa

Huntington's Association of South Africa
Postbox 4640, Tyger Valley, Cape Town 7536, South Africa
Tel: 27-21-9302177; Fax: 27-21-9302178; Mobile: 27-8241 03641
Email: Jschron@iafrica.com

Huntington's United Group South Africa
Mrs Tina-Marie Wessels
Genetic Counselling Clinic
University of the Witwatersrand and the National Health Laboratory Service
Postbox 1038, Johannesburg 2000, South Africa
Tel: 11-489 9243; Fax: 11-489 9226
Email: tina.wessels@nhls.ac.za

Spain

Asociacion de Corea de Huntington Espanola
Fray Junipero Serra 23
08320 El Masnou, Barcelona, Spain
Tel: 34 93 555 3354; Fax: 34-93-555 2130
Email: info@e-huntington.org
Website: http://www.e-huntington.org

Sweden

Huntington Foreningen i Sverige

C/O NHR, Postbox 490 84, 100 28 Stockholm, Sweden

Tel: 46-8-677 7010; Fax: 46-8-24 1 315

Email: nhr@nhr.se; mia.lundstrom@nhr.se

Website: http://www.nhr.se

Switzerland

Schweizerische Huntington Vereinigung

Bahnweg 4, 8156 Oberhasli, Switzerland

Tel: 41-44-885 1941; Fax: 41-44-885 1944; Tel (home): 41-44-885 1942

Email: info@shv.ch

Website: http://www.shv.ch; www.huntington.ch

Turkey

Turkish Huntington Society

Prof. A. Nazli Basak

Bogazici University, Dept of Molecular Biology and Genetics

80815 Bebek, Istanbul, Turkey

Tel: 90-212-359 6679; Fax: 90-212-287 2468

Email: basak@boun.edu.tr

Website: http://www.boun.edu.tr

United Kingdom

England and Wales

Huntington's Disease Association

Downstream Building, 1 London Bridge

London SE1 9BG, United Kingdom

Tel: 44-20-7022 1950; Fax: 44-20-7022 1953

Email: info@hda.org.uk

Website: http://www.hda.org.uk

Scotland

Scottish Huntington's Association

Thistle House, 61 Main Road, Elderslie, Johnstone PA5 9BA, Scotland

Tel: 44-1505-322245; Fax: 44-1505-382980

Email: sha-admin@hdscotland.org

Website: http://www.hdscotland.org

United States of America

Huntington's Disease Society of America

505 Eighth Avenue, Suite 902, New York NY 10018, USA

Tel: 1-212-242 1968; Fax: 1-212-239 3430

Email: hdsainfo@hdsa.org

Website: http://www.hdsa.org

Venezuela

Asociacion Venezolana de Huntington

Mrs Aleska Gonzalez de Zambrano

Av. Principal de Colinas de Bello Monte

Calle Voltaire, Edificio-Palpoc, Piso 4, Apt 41, Parroquia el Recreo

1050 DC Caracas, Venezuela

Tel: 58-212-7517 654; Fax: 58-212-261 5011

Email: avehun@hotmail.com

Other countries

International Huntington Association Office

Gerrit R. Dommerholt

Callunahof 8, 7217 St Harfsen, The Netherlands

Tel: 31-573-431595; Fax: 31-573-431719

Email: iha@huntington-assoc.com; info@huntington-disease.org

Web: http://www.huntington-disease.org; www.huntington-assoc.com

Other organizations

Hereditary Disease Foundation

1427 Seventh Street #22, Santa Monica, CA 90401, USA

Tel: 1-310-450 9913

Email: cures@hdfoundation.org

Website: http://www.hdfoundation.org

International Huntington Association (IHA)

Gerrit R. Dommerholt (Office Manager)

Callunahof 8, 7217 St Harfsen, The Netherlands

Tel: 31-573-431595; Fax: 31-573-431719

Email: iha@huntington-assoc.com; info@huntington-disease.org

Website: http://www.huntington-assoc.com; www.huntington-disease.org

Alliance of Genetic Support Groups

35 Wisconsin Circle, Suite 440, Chevy Chase, MD 20815-7015, USA

Tel: 1-301-652 5553

Email: alliance@capaccess.org

Worldwide Education and Awareness for Movement Disorders (WE MOVE)

One Gustave L. Levy Place, Box 1052, New York, NY 10029, USA

Tel: 1-212-241 8567

Email: wemove@wemove.org

European Federation of Neurological Associations (EFNA)

Viale Pieraccini 6, Firenze 50139, Italy

Tel: 39-055-4362 098; Fax: 39-055-4271 280

Email: efns-branch@pharm.unifi.it

European Organization for Rare Disorders (EURORDIS)

102 Rue Didot, 75014 Paris, France
Tel: 33-1-4416 2747; Fax: 33-1-4416 2712
Email: eurordis@eurordis.org
Website: http://www.eurordis.org

European Huntington Association

Spelonckvaart 30, 9180 Moerbeke-Waas, Belgium
Tel: 32-9-346 8991
Email: bea.deschepper@versateladsl.be
Website: http://www.e-h-a.tripod.com

Euro-HD Network

Tel: 49-731-500 50951
Email: info@euro-hd.net
Website: http://www.euro-hd.net

World Federation of Neurology Research Group on Huntington Disease

Tel: 1-317-274 5742
Email: pconneal@iupui.edu
Website: http://www.wfneurology.org

Huntington Study Group

Tel: 1 310 450 9913
Email: hsgwebmaster@ctcc.rochester.edu
Website: http://www.huntington-study-group.org

The Huntington Project

Tel: 1-585-273 4147
Email: leslie.briner@ctcc.rochester.edu
Website: http://www.huntingtonproject.org

International Huntington Association Contacts

Chile

Dr Marcello Miranda

Llewellyn Jones 1530, Depto 201

Providencia, Santiago, Chile

Tel: 56-2-222 2475; Fax: 56-2-341 1633; Tel (home): 56-2-341 1633

Email: marcelomiranda@terra.cl

China

Mr Yicheng Xu

Beijing, China

Tel: 86-10-6505 1166 ext. 1030; Fax: 86-10-6505 1156

Email: xuyc24@vip.163.com

Egypt

Mr Hany Farid Haleem

6 Omrania Street, Omrania

Giza 12211, Cairo, Egypt

Tel: 202-571 1379

Email: hanyfarid612@yahoo.com

Website: http://www.geocities.com/hd egypt

Hungary

Professor Laszlo Vecsei

Department of Neurology, University of Szeged

Semmelweis Str. 6, H6725 Szeged, Hungary

Tel: 36-62-545351; Fax: 36-62-545 597

Email: vecsei@nepsy.szote.u-szeged.hu

Iran

Mrs Fabiola Hormozain

Email: f-hormozian@yahoo.com

Oman and other African countries

Dr Euan Scrimgeour
Dept of Medicine, College of Medicine, Sultan Qaboos University
Postbox 35, Al-Khod 123, Sultanate of Oman
Tel: 968-513 333; Fax: 968-513 419
Email: scrim@squ.edu.om

Peru

Dr Miriam Velez
Prolongacion
265 Cusco 265, 32 San Miguel, Lima, Peru
Tel: 51-1-328 0504; Tel/Fax (home): 51-1-263 5571
Email: miriamev@yahoo.com

Romania

Dr Florian Alexandru and Maria Magdalena Obretin
Centrul de Recuperare si Reabilitare Neuropsihiatrics
Gura Ocnitei, Ochiuri
Jud. Dambevita, Romania
Tel: 45-4-766-451355
Email: obretin-74@yahoo.com

South Korea

Dr Manho Kim
Dept of Neurology, Seoul National University Hospital
28 Yongondong, Chongnoku
Seoul 110-744, South Korea
Tel: 82-2-760 2193; Fax: 82-2-744 1785
Email: kimmanho@snu.ac.kr

Surinam

Mr Dick IJskes

Paramaribo, Surinam

Email: d.yskes@sr.net

Taiwan

Dr Tso-Ren Wang

Dept of Pediatrics, National Taiwan University Hospital

7 Chung-Sheng S Road, Taipei, Taiwan ROC

Thailand

Dr Siwaporn Chankrachang

Faculty of Medicine, Dept of Neurology, Chiang Mai University

Chiang Mai 50200, Thailand

Tel: 66-53-945 4825; Fax: 66-53-945 481; Mobile: 66-1-6030 555/66-1-8830 303

Email: schankra@mail.med.cmu.ac.th

Uruguay

Mrs Montserrat Martinez

Bvr. Artigas 2087, CP 11800 Montevideo, Uruguay

Tel: 5982-409 8234; Fax: 5982-401 3918

Email: montsemora1954@yahoo.com; lamonse@adinet.com.uy

Zimbabwe

Mr Manu Prajapati

13/23 Rd Ave, Famona Bulawayo, Zimbabwe

Tel: 263-9-64470; Fax: 263-9-883067

Email: tejal@mweb.co.zw

Index